†

C000053195

NIC'S KET(

Author Nicolas Tzenios

Text Johnny Acton, on behalf of Story Terrace

Design Grade Design & Adeline Media, London

Copyright © Nicolas Tzenios

Text is private and confidential

StoryTerrace·

First print October 2018

CONTENTS

FOREWORD

The message of this book can be summed up in one simple sentence:

If you eat sugar you become fat. If you eat fat, you lose weight.

Of course, in practice things aren't quite as simple as this. You have to eat the right kind of fat, in the right quantity and at the right times. It also makes all the difference what else you are putting into your body. The quickest way to become enormous, for example, is to consume high quantities of both fat and carbohydrate, as found in the worst and hardest to resist doughnut. But the basic message remains true. It isn't fat that's responsible for the epidemic of obesity sweeping the planet. It's sugar!

Intuitively, it sounds crazy to suggest that the way to lose body fat is to eat more fat than you are already doing. But remember, biology is not simple mathematics or physics. Our bodies break down what we eat and turn it into other things, including energy.

INTRODUCTION

As you will discover as you read this book, I am very fond of doing medical tests on myself. In fact, it's one of my defining characteristics.

A few months ago, I noticed that my cholesterol readings were getting higher. By this stage, I had been on my own version of the keto diet, a low carb, high fat regime that is the subject of this book, for more than a year.

So, my cholesterol was elevated, but I also discovered that I had extremely low levels of something called C-reactive protein in my blood. This is a substance produced by the liver in response to inflammation in the body. High scores are associated with increased risk of stroke or heart attack, because these conditions usually start with inflammation in the blood circulation system. Before I went on the keto diet, my C-protein score was around 4. Now it was down to 0.4.

In conventional terms, this was puzzling. Other things being equal, you'd expect a high cholesterol reading, like a high C-protein score, to point to a heightened chance of stroke or heart attack. But my C-protein score suggested exactly the opposite.

I went to my (long-suffering!) doctor, who was intrigued. Neither he nor I was particularly surprised by the high cholesterol score, as eating fat and breaking it down, which are central to the keto diet, inevitably mean that you have a lot of the stuff in your blood. But he gave me a more sophisticated test to find out more. It showed that my level of HDL – high density lipoprotein, often described as 'good' cholesterol – was normal, and my triglycerides – a type of fat present in the blood - were very low. But my LDLs – low density lipoprotein, also known as 'bad cholesterol' – were off the scale.

Too much LDL in the blood can lead to a build-up of what is known as plaque on their walls. It is made up of cholesterol, calcium and other substances, and is undesirable at the best of times because it narrows the arteries, allowing less blood to pass through. What is really bad news, though, is plates of plaque breaking away from the arterial walls. They form lumps in the blood that can cause strokes or heart attacks.

When he saw how high my LDL levels were, my doctor suggested I do another test to determine exactly what was going on in my arteries. This was the PLAC® test, which measures the levels of an enzyme called lipoprotein phospholipase. This is produced by the body in response to excessive levels of LDL. Unfortunately, the enzyme itself causes problems, triggering a chain of events which end up causing a pathological abnormality in the walls of the blood vessels. This sets the stage for atherosclerosis, plaque accumulation and rupture.

When I left the consulting room, my doctor said, "take care". I could see in his face that he was a bit worried. My wife wasn't too happy either, to say the least, when I told her about the test. Then I got an email from the person who had analysed the results. It said, "You're not just at risk, you're at very high risk". The message was essentially "Start saying your prayers".

Now I was starting to get worried too. But my scientific brain told me that in order to have detached plaque, there needed to be inflammation at the release site. If this was happening in my body I would have a high C-protein score but in fact I had a very low one. Something wasn't adding up.

I was due to travel to Belgium, where I have a Lebanese friend who is a magnificent heart doctor. I arranged to see him, hoping he would give me a referral letter for a 3-D heart test. I didn't tell him about the plaque result at first because I didn't want to prejudice his examination of me. He did an echo doppler test and said "You've got a magnificent heart. Why did you want this test?" So, I told him. He immediately ordered me to get back on the bed and got to work on me. He couldn't find any plaque plates anywhere but told me I needed to do a more sophisticated test, which was why I'd gone to see him in the first place.

By this stage, my wife was desperately trying to pull words out of his mouth. "Tell him eating fat is bad", she implored him. "Tell him!" Turning to me, he said "I've never heard that people can eat a high fat diet and be healthy." "When did you last read a book about food?", I asked him. He had no real answer to this. He just advised me to stop my high-intensity training and gave me my referral letter.

At the time, my exercise program was getting my pulse rate up to 190 or higher every day. I was pretty sure that if there was a serious problem, my heart would have failed by now. But I wasn't 100% certain and I'm not a suicidal guy, so I went along with his advice for a few days. I also made sure my life insurance was up to date.

The Belgians told me it would be three weeks before I could have the 3-D heart scan. I didn't want to delay for that long, so I called a friend in Germany. "Come here and we'll do the test immediately", he said. So, I headed for Aachen. The technician who administered the test said, "I'm not a doctor but everything looks very good to me".

They were looking for two things. The first was my calcium score. When the results came back, they showed a calcification of zero – perfection. The second was visual evidence of blockage or damage to the veins or arteries. They couldn't find any. In other words, the plaque reading had been rubbish. My friend told me I had the heart of an extremely healthy 18-year-old.

I still don't have a certain answer to the riddle of the misleading plaque result, but I think something must have been circulating in my blood as a result of my keto diet that the test mistook for plaque. I have asked my doctor in the UK to write to his colleagues telling them not to take the plaque test too seriously for people who are on keto diets.

Obviously, it was a great relief to find that I wasn't in mortal peril after all, but there was more to my satisfaction than that. I soon realised that what we had discovered had struck a blow against the prevailing medical wisdom. "Man", I said to myself, "old dietary medicine died today. And so did old nutrition". It quickly became clear to me that I needed to speak out and let the world know that there was another way to live.

This 'other way' has nothing to do with the tasteless, low fat, carb-infested items that fill the supermarket shelves, and even the shop at your gym. For years, marketing men in league with the old medicine guys have been trying to sell you high-carb chocolate bars by adding a few nuts and branding them as high protein. No. Enough. Eat fat and enjoy it. Luxuriate in the richness of full fat double cream. But eat it without sugars, either direct ones or hidden ones. There are no such things as healthy sugars. The two words just don't go together.

Like the results of my 3-D heart scan after that plaque test, the keto diet challenges some of the most basic assumptions of nutritional science. But as I mean to show you, many of those assumptions are wrong. Not just wrong but extremely harmful. This is because they support a diet that is doing terrible damage to the health of billions.

I don't expect you to swallow this idea easily. It would be

strange if you did, because our dietary indoctrination goes very deep indeed. "Eating fat is bad for you". "If you don't eat lots of fruit you'll die". "If you don't eat anything at all for 20 hours, you'll go the same way, or at best you'll be weak and depleted". We can all relate to these attitudes. After all, they have had the weight of official, government science behind them for many decades. They have also become central to the way our economy and food culture works, and people don't like change. But they don't like being obese or diabetic either. And the public health costs of our 'old' ideas about food are simply too big to ignore.

Don't worry, I won't be attempting to bamboozle you with science (although I will try to back up my claims with references to respectable studies). That can come later, for those who are interested or need to know. This is a book aimed squarely at laypersons, particularly those who make the decisions about health policy that influence all our lives.

1

PART ONE – ME

My Story

My name is Nicolas. I'm a 47-year-old education-focused business manager, and I have been a university and hospital administrator for many years. I'm unusual in some ways. For a real treat, I nibble on a lump of butter. But 18 months ago I was enormous. Now I'm slim, fit and happy.

I was born in Beirut in 1971, the eldest of four siblings. My father's family were originally Greek, but they fled from what used to be called the Ottoman Empire in the 1900s. My mother was Lebanese. When I was a baby, I used to cry and cry until she gave me another feed. From the start, I had double doses of food.

My mother was always opposed to food with anything added, including sugar. She prepared all our food at home to avoid the harmful effect of industrial packaged sweets and treats. But I still got chubby. I lost weight during puberty but

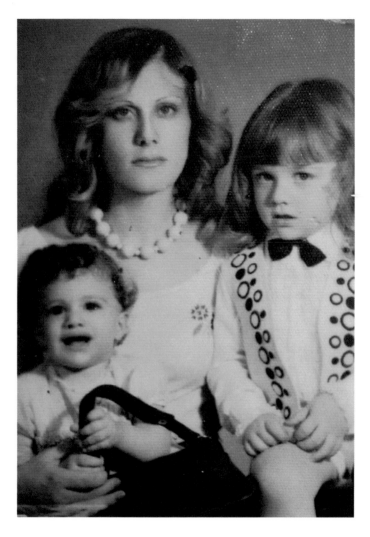

The blonde boy is me at two years old with my wonderful mum and my sister who was to become a doctor

that was due to hormonal factors. I soon started putting it back on again.

Most of the people on my father's side of the family are big. I have one cousin who is so fat he can't freely walk. I seem to have inherited a predisposition in this direction.

When I was four, civil war broke out in Lebanon. Life was very hard. We happened to live in the mainly Muslim part of town, where my family had its furniture business.

The one thing my parents were determined to do despite the war was get me into the best school possible. I got a place at Notre Dame de Jamhour, a Roman Catholic school which was attended by most of the top French-speaking people in Beirut. I am still very grateful to the Jesuits who ran it. They anchored in me the principles I have needed for a successful life, based on believing in God and doing my best.

To get there, sometimes we had to pass under bullets being fired on the crossings between the Muslim quarter and the Christian section, where the school was located. But my father was insistent, even when the fighting was at its most extreme. "Without a good education, your life won't be worth living", he said. In my mother's philosophy, the words "a good education" were topped with "living as a good Christian and a disciplined person".

The main thing my parents agreed on was the importance of their children pursuing careers in medicine. My sisters were certainly convinced: the elder one is a gynaecologist, married to a radiologist, while the younger one is a child psychologist,

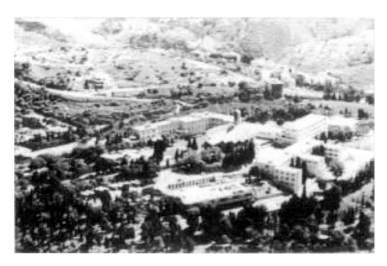

Notre Dame de Jamhour

married to a surgeon. I too am completely fascinated by medicine – I read about it every day – and I believe that becoming a doctor is the highest calling to which a person can aspire (apart from becoming a priest - a doctor of souls - which clearly isn't for everyone). I started a pre-medical course in biology at the Lebanese American University of Lebanon, as well as a preparatory course for studying Medicine in Cyprus, then enrolled in a language course to enable me to study Medicine in Russia. But in the end I decided that 10 years of training was too long for me. I wanted to start earning money as soon as possible. So, in the embraces of fast-changing Russia, I skipped the medical course that I had planned to attend there and enrolled in a distance business studies course.

My parents were extremely disappointed by my decision not to train as a doctor. They were even more disappointed when I told them I had met someone and that we were going to get married. I'll never forget the letter I received back from them. They had censored out my wife's name in black ink. "You're too young to get married", they said. "If you insist on doing this, you'll get no help from us. You'll have to survive on your own". (Thankfully, through God's blessings, my mother's prayers and my wife's unending support, I thrived and survived, and my wife became one of my parents' favourite people).

When my parents said, "If you get married, you're on your own", it triggered something in me. I felt I had to prove to myself that I wasn't dependent on anything external, except for God. Addictive foods definitely fitted into this category. I felt I needed to give them up for the self-discipline.

As far as I'm concerned, you can learn discipline from your parents, the army, the church or in many other ways. The important thing is that you learn it from somewhere. Personally, I learned it from the Jesuits at my school and from my mother. Now the time had come to put it into practice.

At that stage, I wasn't a church goer. Between the ages of about 17 and 20, I had a kind of revolt against the Church and all rules that I felt were made by man rather than God. But I had seen my Catholic friends fasting at school and my Christian Orthodox mother doing it at home, so I decided I would do the Lent fast.

I gave up meat and fish and when Easter came, I continued to do without them. I also gave up alcohol, smoking, coffee, strawberries, bananas and anything else that I liked that wasn't absolutely necessary. I didn't feel proud, just better about myself and healthier.

Anyway, when I received that letter from my parents, I sold my leather jacket and used the money to buy two rings and pay a month's rent on our apartment. Then a miracle happened. I met someone who I was able to do a deal with that earned me $50,000 in a couple of weeks (fully legally, in case you have any doubts). This enabled me to pay for the distance learning course in international law and business that I had signed up for at an American university in Moscow.

Someone or something evidently wanted to help me along the path I had chosen, because before long I was introduced to the president of the Medical University in Kursk, a man who was clearly open to new ideas. He told me that the university was experiencing a significant budget shortfall. Shortly afterwards, on a trip home to the Lebanon, I chanced upon the perfect way for him to make up the deficit.

At the time, my sister was finishing off her MCAT – a qualification designed to get people into med school – as were most of her friends. They were all depressed, because the political situation in Lebanon, which was then under Syrian domination, meant that only those with unusually good connections could get university places. Here were all these smart, ambitious young people with no way of continuing their medical education.

Suddenly, a thought occurred to me. Russia had some of best medical teaching programs in the world and had been always very welcoming of foreign students. If Kursk Medical University could offer affordable training in English, I bet my sister and her friends would be prepared to go there to study. I was also sure that there would be thousands of candidates from other countries willing to do the same. The key would be for the courses to be taught in English. I knew the medicine at Kursk was excellent, but I also knew that foreign students were reluctant to study in any language other than English, because it was difficult then to pass the exams necessary to practice in English-speaking countries.

As soon as I got back to Russia, I went to see the president of the university. "If I help you teach medicine in English", I asked him, "will you hire me?". "Yes" he said, without a moment's hesitation. I was now vice president of a medical university at the age of only 24. My parents weren't disappointed anymore!

For the next ten years, I travelled around the world drumming up business for the medical university. The first batch of foreign students were Lebanese. The next wave came from Malaysia, after we successfully lobbied the local authorities to accept medical degrees from Kursk. They were followed by students from Commonwealth nations. Today, Kursk is the top medical university in Russia.

When I lived in Russia during the 1990s, I lost weight at first because I was not used to the taste of the food (I highly appreciate it now). But gradually I began to enjoy it, and started piling on the pounds. With hindsight, this wasn't very surprising. The local diet was extremely high in carbohydrates. It was all cream, bread and potatoes (no meat as I was beginning my journey as a vegetarian). I was a vegetarian for 18 years and a vegan for most of the lent days during that period. I didn't drink alcohol, coffee or tea, and I didn't smoke. But I still got very fat.

In 2004 my mother got sick, so I went back home to Lebanon to be with her. At this stage, I weighed around 100kg/220lbs. One day, my father, who never made dramatic gestures, suddenly left the table in the middle of a family meal. "I will not sit and watch you eat yourself to death", he announced.

This shook me up so much that I made up a pretty drastic diet, which wasn't keto (which I hadn't heard about yet), but did have some of its features. It was low carb, low fat and no grains, but I did eat peas and beans, which are high in sugar. I also got through about a kilo/2.2lbs of cucumbers per day.

I did lose weight but there were no spiritual benefits, which I would later discover to be one of the best things about keto. My head didn't feel any nicer or clearer. And the regime was very hard to maintain. Sugar and fat are the two most satisfying eating experiences life has to offer, and while it's OK to do without one of them, to forsake both is a big ask. It's just too miserable. So, I slipped.

While I was in Lebanon, I opened a few clinics. This was very stressful. When you are stressed out, your system produces high levels of cortisol. This is the 'fight or flight' hormone. It interferes with the process of your body burning off fat. "This is an emergency and you may need it", it tells it, "so don't use it – store it". As a result, I started putting on weight again, in spite of my diet.

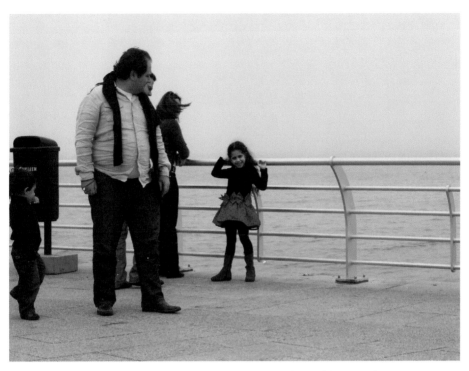

After gaining weight following the cucumber diet (with my nephews)

When I moved to London at the end of this period, I was around 93kg. At first, I walked five or six miles a day, which helped keep the weight gain in check. But after a while I stopped - it isn't easy dragging tens of extra kilograms around with you. Then the inevitable happened: I began to balloon.

One day, I went to church and met my uncle there. He took a long hard look at me – by now I was 112kg – and said "Nicolas, this isn't good". Then he told me about a doctor friend of his who fed his obese patients through tubes in their noses. Apparently, they would lose ten per cent of their body weight in the course of ten days. I couldn't bring myself to sign up for this, but the very fact that my uncle was suggesting

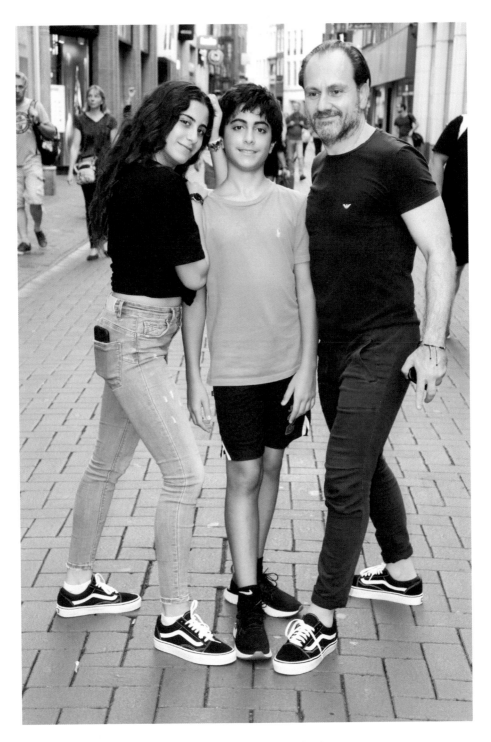

With the same nephews after keto

it made me realise that the time had come to do something drastic. So, I decided to do the Atkins diet, which was big news at the time. It has various phases but essentially it is low-carb, high protein and high fat.

"Bless Doctor Atkins", I always say. As we shall see, he was a visionary who set a trend for all of us. He didn't fully understand his own diet – in particular, he failed to realise that much of the excess protein we consume ends up being converted to body fat anyway, while encouraging his followers to eat a lot of protein - but he was the inspiration for so many people and paved the way for the keto revolution.

Using his method, I got my weight down to 82-83kg. Unfortunately, this turned out to be an unbreakable ceiling, or perhaps it would be more accurate to call it a floor. It was incredibly frustrating to see the scales stuck at the 82kg mark. I even bought another set in the hope that this would make a difference, but it wasn't the scales that were to blame. It was excess protein.

To my dismay, my weight eventually started increasing, although I was continuing to follow the Atkins diet, consuming lots of protein and very little carbohydrate. After a year, I was back up to 101kg. I was starting to run out of ideas.

Lent is a big deal to Orthodox people like me and it is a period when we are expected to make changes to our diets. A few days before Lent 2017, I said to myself "OK, no more Atkins. I'll eat what I want for three days, then I'll work out what to do for my Lenten fast". I was in Belgium at the time, so there were lots of good Michelin-starred restaurants!

Over the weekend, I spoke to my nephew in Canada on the telephone. He told me about some body builders at his gym who somehow managed to burn off all their body fat ahead of competitions. Not surprisingly, given my weight predicament, I wondered how they did it. He said it had to do with something called 'macros'.

I was intrigued and did some searching on the internet. It turned out that 'macros' was short for 'macronutrients'. It denotes the three main calorie producing food groups: protein, fat and carbohydrate. 'Doing your macros' is working out how much of each you should be eating every day to obtain a specific result, for example losing a certain amount of weight in a given time period. To discover the answer, you need to use a 'macro calculator'. I found one online and typed in my numbers. What I didn't realise at the time was that the macro calculator I was using was specially designed for a keto diet. I just got lucky! Anyway, it told me I should be eating more fat. I decided to give it a try.

Being a religious man, I went to see my priest, who I saw as my spiritual father, to tell him about what I was proposing to do. It was basically the opposite of the traditional Orthodox Lenten fast, which is all about eating bread and potatoes and cutting out all meat, fish, eggs, dairy and things like olive oil. (In fact, it's virtually an all-carbs diet, if you leave out the protein from the beans which you are encouraged to eat.) But as far as I'm concerned, the point of the fast is self-discipline, not some peculiar aversion God has to certain foods. He doesn't need us to give up eggs for himself! What I was planning was certainly going to require discipline. So I said "Father, I need your blessing to do my fast eating fish" (adding "and maybe eggs" in a very low voice, but in fact I didn't eat any during the Lent period). And he said "OK".

On day one, I cooked up a big soup with fish and greens. I mostly ate the liquid, along with just a little of the residue. I felt pretty hungry, to be honest, so I borrowed my wife's vape to occupy my mouth. I also took the dog for a walk and felt unusually tired afterwards.

On day two, my spirits were low. I didn't know about MCTs at the time, which would have made life much easier (there'll be more about these later), but I did put some coconut oil in my coffee. This helped a bit but I felt faint when I stood up. From past experience, I knew this meant my blood sugar was probably out of kilter, so I bought a machine to monitor it. I found that my sugar level was indeed fluctuating quite a lot, but my doctor told me that was to be expected given the change in my diet, so I wasn't unduly alarmed.

The next day, I bought two portions of sashimi and wolfed them down. I repeated this purchase on day four, but this time I felt full after the first helping and didn't eat the other one. This was the first sign my appetite was adjusting to the new diet.

At some point in the first few days, I took the dog for a walk and when he started running, I found myself doing the same thing. This was very unusual for me at the time. I went home, measured my blood sugar and found it was lower than normal. Then I went for another run with the dog. Suddenly, I felt a flash of heat in my head. "Oh no", I said to myself, "something bad has happened here". Now, when I tested my blood, the sugar reading was very high. What had happened, I decided, was that my insulin system had responded to the running by saying to my liver "go and get us some sugar from Nic's muscles to help us deal with this unusual situation".

In Belgium, it was difficult to acquire a machine to measure the levels of ketones in my blood, but I realised that's what I needed to do. My first reading was 0.6. The next day it had risen to 1.0. Soon it settled into the desirable range of between 1.5 and 3.0, though sometimes nowadays, as a result of the intermittent fasting I have added to my regime (more on this later), it goes to 4.0 or above.

I would advise anyone doing my diet to buy a blood ketone measuring machine. There is information about the options available on page 121. For the diet to be successful, it is absolutely essential to know whether you are in ketosis – the state in which your body is using fat rather than glucose as its fuel. That way, you can make appropriate adjustments to your intake of food if you are not. You will know that you are in ketosis if you can smell acetone on your breath (this is the substance that gives nail varnish its distinctive odour), but a machine gives you a precise reading, which is invaluable. It is possible to measure your ketones by testing your urine, but blood samples work best. You just need to make a tiny prick in one of your fingers. You soon get used to it. People with diabetes have to do it all the time.

In next to no time, I was losing weight consistently. This made me very happy, especially as I wasn't feeling hungry or deprived. After Lent, I started eating meat again, and this halted the weight loss until I spotted I was overdoing the steaks. Today, I understand that you should stick to no more than 160g/6 oz per meal and 320g/12 oz per day. As we will see, Dr Atkins' big mistake was not realising the extent to which excess protein gets turned into stored fat. I switched to fish and found that the pounds started falling off again, but eating fish made me feel hungry and I had had enough of it (I had eaten loads of it for two years while I was transitioning from vegetarian to a meat eater). So, I eventually went back to meat, but not too much of it.

Since I started my keto diet, I have lost 32kg/88lbs, on top of the 12kg compared to my peak that I had already shed when I began it. All of this has been fat, and I have even gained some muscle due to exercise. I feel energised and happy and can do ten times more work than before. My biological age, according to a machine I use at the gym, is 32 – 15 years less than my actual one.

Why Listen to Me?

There is no shortage of books about the keto diet out there. Why, you may very reasonably be asking yourself, does the world need another one? More to the point, why does it need this specific one?

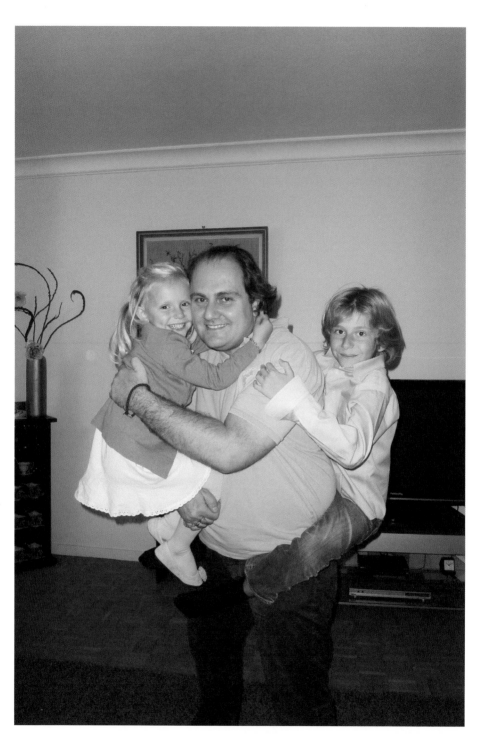

Before my Atkins

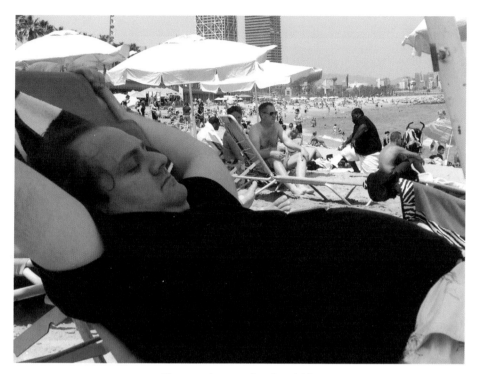

After starting to gain after Atkins

My first answer is that this is more than just a diet book. It is a call to the people who make the decisions that determine our collective attitudes to food to question everything they think they know about the subject. It seeks profound social change. The reason is simple: the received wisdom about diet is damaging lives. Not just millions of them, but billions. And this is a problem we can do something about.

Nevertheless, the question remains, why listen to me? Here are some of the reasons why I believe you should:

i) I have tried this diet on myself. I know it works. I'm not just some academic doctor trying his theories out on other people.

ii) What makes me 'special' is my extraordinary track record of doing medical tests on myself (well, other people find it extraordinary). I have conducted more than 3,000 of them. People say, "but you don't have a medical degree". My answer is that all the tests I have done on myself are my executive medical degree. I have an unrivalled first-hand knowledge of the effects of eating specific foods in specific quantities.

Some people might call me obsessive but as far as I'm concerned, the only thing I'm obsessed with is finding the truth. I have experimented with the effects of eating all kinds of food, and I am scientifically minded enough to change only one variable at a time, so the results are trustworthy. And I truly enjoy the process. Knowledge makes me euphoric. Every time I learn something new, I feel I have accomplished something.

iii) I was vice president of a medical university for many years. I have run several clinics and hospitals and am always spending time with doctors, not least the ones in my family. I therefore know how the system works and am in a position to understand it.

Over the past 18 months, I have struggled with doctors,

arguing my case and sticking to my guns despite considerable scepticism. "You are starving yourself", they all said. "You'll get sick. Your cholesterol will get too high and you will kill yourself". Well, I've proved some of them wrong and some of them are starting to admit it.

I am not against doctors. Far from it. I consider theirs to be the most noble profession in the world and my entire life is devoted to medicine. But as with any job, there are good doctors and less good ones. Part of the problem is that they are usually so busy they have no time to read and update their knowledge. I strongly advise anyone taking up my diet to enlist the help and support of their doctor, but they need to be aware that there is likely to be some resistance because of what they will have been taught in med school.

iv) Everything I say is correlated with studies, particularly 'meta' ones (studies of studies).

v) As part of my ongoing PhD study (see page 107), I will be conducting original clinical research into the effect of my diet on telomeres. These are strands of DNA at the end of our chromosomes that protect them from damage. The longer they are, the healthier we are. Crucially, they can change in response to changes in our lifestyle. If we can prove that Nic's Keto Diet increases the length of the telomeres of the participants in the study, and I am very confident that we can, we will have objective evidence of its health benefits.

vi) My practical religious background (mainly influenced by strict Orthodox fasting practices) gives me an angle on fasting that is different from what you are likely to encounter elsewhere.

Religion is very important to me. I was brought up Greek Orthodox, studied for 12 years in a Catholic Jesuit school and am now a reader in the Russian Orthodox Church. One of the biggest features of the Orthodox religion is fasting. In fact, I have calculated that there are more than hundreds of days of the year in which members of the church are supposed to be refrain from eating at least some foods! Nevertheless, the Orthodox definition of fasting is not the same as my own. To me, fasting means not eating at all. Maybe this was true within all religions until they made modifications to fit in with the practicalities of life.

Fasting, (the easy, intermittent kind) is a very important part of my diet, and you will find information about its role in various religious traditions in Appendix 4. What I will say for now is that growing up Orthodox accustomed me from a young age to paying attention to what I ate and being disciplined about it. To that you can add 16 years of veganism, which required me to check every small detail of what the food I ate contained and how it was prepared.

vii) I'm a man on a mission (see next page).

My Mission

I believe that for more than 40 years, we have been sold a lie about diet.

As somebody immersed in the world of medicine, I have a powerful desire to help overturn society's misguided nutritional assumptions. I also feel that I have a duty to share what I have learned.

I wouldn't be writing this book if it was just about losing weight. I think I have an obligation to every human being to tell the other side of the story. This is the health dimension. It is all about our addiction to sugars - invisible sugars in the blood. They are in milk and even in fruit. And they are killing people every day. Yet we aren't saying anything about it.

There is amazing work being done out there which hasn't yet been widely reported. If my small, very humble book can attract a few more people to the keto diet, writing it will have been worthwhile.

But I'm not a crusader. They tend to get killed and turned into martyrs. You need to survive to continue the fight. In any case, I have spent too much time in medical circles to accept some of the more extravagant claims made for keto diets. As you will see, I am not convinced, for example, that they are the 'solution' to cancer. I am, however, quite sure that keto can cure type 2 diabetes and help enormously with epilepsy, Parkinson's disease and polycystic ovary syndrome. And I am beyond certain that it can improve your life more than you can imagine.

I see my mission as having two parts. The first is a technical challenge: showing people how to lose weight and become healthier and happier. The second part is the adaptive challenge of changing mentalities. This is the subject of Part Four of this book.

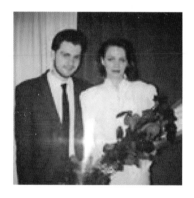

Just lost weight before my marriage in April 1992

2

PART TWO – THE SCIENCE

Insulin Resistance: The Core of the Problem

An important premise of the keto approach is that the real problem with the 'modern' diet is what it does to our hormones. These are the substances, secreted into the blood by our glands, that regulate and control the activity of our cells and organs.

Addiction to sugar and carbohydrates has messed up one hormone in particular, with devastating consequences: Insulin. Produced by the pancreas, it plays a vital role in the regulation of the amount of sugar in your blood. Insulin resistance occurs when the cells in the body no longer respond to the hormone properly. The result is that blood sugar stays excessively high all or most of the time. Eventually, this can cause type 2 diabetes. It is also a major cause of obesity.

The laws of physics don't operate in a straightforward way in human biology. For many years, we have been trying to apply them to diet, assuming for example that "calories in means calories out" (in other words, eating them will make you fat). But – and it's hard to overstate the importance of this – to look at things this way is to ignore hormonal factors. And it is hormones that determine how you metabolise your food. Sure, there's some truth in the old idea that "you are what you eat". If you consume rubbish, you're likely to be unhealthy. Indeed, this is one of the cornerstones of my keto diet. But it's important not to take the idea too literally. Nobody seriously believes that if you eat a lot of avocado you'll turn into one.

So, the way in which your body processes food is controlled by your hormones. What makes things complicated is the fact that the food you eat influences your hormones. They don't just govern how our bodies respond to our diets; they respond to them. It's as if the efficiency of the thermostat which controls the temperature in your house was influenced by how hot it is!

We can only cope with about 4g/1/7oz of sugar in our bloodstreams. If the level rises any higher than this, it needs to be converted into something else. The body's first port of call is to turn the sugar into glycogen, which is the form in which it stores glucose as fuel. But we can only store about 0.6kg/1.25lbs of glycogen, mainly in our livers and muscles. Once this capacity is reached, our bodies start to convert blood sugar into fat. Insulin is the hormone that governs both these processes. It tells the liver when to start synthesising glycogen, and it tells the body's so-called adipose cells when to start absorbing lipids (fats). No prizes for guessing what happens when the latter happens to excess. We get fat.

The pancreas will desperately pump out insulin to ensure that our blood sugar level stays within acceptable levels. If it has to do this routinely, we run the risk of developing insulin resistance. This can cause us to become pre-diabetic or to contract full-on type 2 diabetes, not to mention becoming obese.

The way to prevent this happening is to avoid insulin spikes. When we eat certain foods, our insulin levels rise rapidly, causing the body to burn up the glucose in the blood very quickly. This has two main effects. It causes a condition called hypoglycaemia, the symptoms of which include dizziness, sweating and shaking, and ultimately seizures or a coma. It also jolts the body into fat absorption mode, causing you to put on weight.

If insulin is injected into a person's body, there can be an alarming build-up of fat around the injection site., as the photo below shows. If this doesn't convince you that too much of the stuff can cause weight gain, I don't know what will:

Fat doesn't cause insulin spikes.

Protein spikes your insulin a bit.

Carbohydrates, particularly sugar, spike it a lot.

Slow sugars, for instance the ones found in soluble fibre, do this less than 'fast' ones like sucrose and fructose, but the effect lasts for longer.

Insulin resistance tends to cause a further problem, which is resistance to leptin, the hormone that tells you when you are full. In simple terms, the hunger that insulin resistance promotes overrides the leptin response, so you don't feel full even when you've eaten enough.

It is almost impossible to eat less while continuing to eat carbohydrates, because the insulin spikes this causes are essentially instructions to the body to consume more food (and to ignore the feedback provided by leptin, which is telling you to stop). In theory, you could restrict yourself to 1200 calories a day and allow yourself to obtain some of these through eating bread, but you would be stoking the fires and fighting your physiology. Bread, potatoes and so on just make you want to eat more. Fruit juice is even worse.

I've cheated on my diet once or twice and found that putting something sweet in my mouth is like giving a drink to an alcoholic. I start to crave more. Recently, I went through passport control at Nice airport and found there was nowhere to eat except Starbucks. I had a cookie and before I knew it I'd eaten every sweet thing there.

Using artificial sweeteners is problematic, because they have a similar effect. Some of them actually cause insulin spikes, and even the ones that don't, like monk fruit, tend to make you crave food by association.

The way to control your hunger is not to eat sweet things.

GLUCAGON: YOUR FRIENDLY HORMONE

Insulin is not the only hormone produced by the pancreas. The same organ also generates Glucagon, which in many ways is the complete opposite. The two hormones work in tandem in what is known as a 'negative feedback loop' to keep the amount of sugar in the blood at a safe level.

Insulin is released when blood glucose levels are high. It tells the cells in your body to take in glucose from the bloodstream. They then either use it immediately as fuel, convert it into glycogen to be stored in the liver or muscles, or convert it into lipids to be stored as fat.

Glucagon, by contrast, is released when blood glucose levels are low, or when the body needs additional glucose in response to vigorous exercise. It tells the liver and muscles to convert the glycogen stored within them back into glucose, to provide the body with fuel.

Glucagon also plays an important role in two other processes. The first is the activation of gluconeogenesis, through which amino acids are converted into glucose (see page 47). The second is the breaking down of stored body fat (triglycerides) into fatty acids, which the cells of the body can then use as fuel. This is what ketosis is all about.

To put it in simple terms, when you eat food that causes the pancreas to produce insulin, you are not benefiting from the action of Glucagon. On the keto diet, Glucagon is very much your friend.

How the Human Diet Has Changed Over Time

Life was precarious for our hunter-gatherer ancestors, so when they ate they needed to store any sources of energy in excess of their immediate needs in their bodies for later use. Insulin enabled them to do this. It also allowed them to convert excess protein into energy stores via the process of gluconeogenesis (see page 47). This was particularly important when our forebears made a kill, as they would consume much more protein in a single sitting than we typically do nowadays.

In some ways, the problems began with the domestication of grains around 10,000 years ago. People found themselves eating far more carbohydrates than their bodies had evolved to expect, putting strain on their systems. What really sent the situation into overdrive, though, was the invention of refined sugar. In the Middle Ages, this was a luxury, and more expensive in real terms than cocaine is today, but by the eighteenth century it began to become affordable to ordinary people. As more and more of it was consumed over time, diseases like diabetes, arteriosclerosis and obesity began to proliferate. When high fructose corn syrup was introduced in the 1970s, things got even worse.

We have been boiling in sugar from a long time, but like the proverbial crab in the gradually heated saucepan, we haven't noticed what has been happening to us. Yes, people are living longer now. This is largely a consequence of us having become so good at preventing and curing infection diseases. But this may not remain the case for long, owing to our abuse of antibiotics both in our own bodies and those of domesticated animals. In the meantime, 'lifestyle' diseases are rampant.

The potential solution – keto science – has been around for much longer than you might think. In 1862, a 66-year-old undertaker named William Banting went to see an ear, nose and throat specialist named Dr William Harvey, complaining that he was having hearing problems. Harvey diagnosed that his problem wasn't deafness, it was obesity. Banting had so much body fat that some of it was pressing on his inner ear. Harvey instructed him to give up starch, sugar, potatoes and beer.

12 months later, Banting had shed three stone (almost 20kg). His ear problem had vanished, and he felt fantastic. He decided to write a book about the diet called *Letter on Corpulence*. It sold 63,000 copies, a fantastic number at the time, and the word 'bant' entered the English language as a verb meaning 'to diet'.

Keto proper was introduced by Dr Russell Wilder of the prestigious Mayo Clinic in Minnesota in the early 1920s. He developed a low carbohydrate diet for epileptic children, and found it to be highly effective. Now we have discovered that his approach has a far wider application than he can have imagined. In fact, almost everyone can benefit from it.

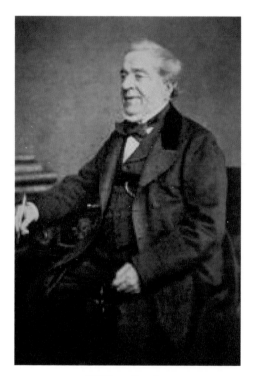

William Banting

The Costly Error: Ancel Keys and the Demonisation of Fat

During the 1950s, Americans started to become alarmed at increasing rates of heart disease among business executives. This was puzzling, because on paper these were some of the best fed people in the world.

A professor of physiology at the University of Minnesota named Ancel Keys was certain he had found the culprit. It was cholesterol, particularly saturated fat. He persuaded America's most prominent cardiologist Dr Paul White, and the pair presented their findings at the International Society of Cardiology's congress in Washington in 1954. Soon after this, Newsweek magazine ran an influential article headlined 'Fat's the villain'.

The following year, President Eisenhower had a heart attack. Interest in the cardiovascular epidemic went into overdrive, as did the search for a solution.

To prove his hypothesis, Keys began his notorious Seven Countries Study. Armed with a blood cholesterol measuring machine, he tested almost 13,000 men in Greece, Italy, the USA, the Netherlands, Japan, and Finland between 1958 and 1964. His findings were unambiguous: coronary heart disease and strokes were directly correlated with high blood cholesterol.

There were two major problems with Keys's methodology. First, he made the logical and factual error of assuming that high fat in the blood was caused by high fat in the diet. Second, he cherry-picked the nations to fit his theory. He ignored countries like Germany and France, which had high rates of saturated fat consumption and low incidences of heart disease. When confronted with evidence of other populations with these characteristics, like Swiss Alpine farmers or the Maasi herders of East Africa, he said they had "no relevance".

In time, Keys's hypothesis was adopted by the American Heart Association and influential health organisations all over the world. Not surprisingly, businesses seized on the opportunity to promote their products as low-fat, while lacing them with sugar.

The idea of fat as the enemy has penetrated our society so deeply that people are only beginning to question it. Yet it rests on some very dubious science indeed.

What is Ketosis?

In order to live, our bodies need to generate energy.

When we eat carbohydrates, the body converts them into a simple sugar called glucose. Some of this is used immediately by the cells.

Ketosis is the state in which the body is burning fat rather than glucose as its primary fuel. Our bodies are designed to be able to do this. In fact, it is worth asking why it is that we can only store about 2000 calories of glucose, but many thousands of calories-worth of fat. The answer is that fat is a safer source of energy and one that our bodies are positively expecting to use.

Sugar does have some important functions. Your brain requires glucose to function properly, but very, very little, and you have reserves in your muscles. You DO need sugar for the optimum delivery of immediate energy, and I certainly wouldn't advise Tour de France racers to stick to a keto diet before heading up Mont Ventoux. But for normal life, including what you might call mental uphill races, ketones are enough. In fact, they're better than that. In many ways, you function much better in ketosis than when your body is being powered by glucose.

The body can run on either carbohydrates or fat, but other things being equal it will turn to the carbs first. Essentially, if you are on a high carbohydrate diet, your body gets very lazy about burning fat. It will only start to do this when you don't consume enough carbs to meet your energy needs, and when you've exhausted your glycogen supplies.

Eating fat will provide your system with fuel and acclimatise it to relying on this alternative energy source, but if you want to start shedding body fat, you will obviously need to leave the body with a shortfall. Only when it has exhausted the carbs you eat, your stores of glycogen and the fat in your diet will your system start burning up your body fat.

Ketosis should not be confused with ketoacidosis, a potentially life-threatening condition that can afflict people with type 1 diabetes. Both are associated with an increase in the levels of ketones in the blood, but in ketoacidosis, these have got dangerously out of hand. In 'normal' people, insulin acts to keep the production of ketones within safe levels. If they rise too high, the insulin tells the body to switch to glucose/glycogen. Type 1 diabetics, whose bodies cannot produce insulin, do not have access to this correction process.

A person in ketosis is likely to have a ketone score of between 1 and 3 millimoles per litre. In a person with ketoacidosis, it will rise to 15 or more.

WHAT ARE KETONE BODIES?

Ketone bodies are water-soluble molecules manufactured by the liver from fatty acids. This happens when there is not enough insulin in the blood to enable the body to use glucose as its primary source of energy. The liver then instructs adipose cells to release the fatty acids they are storing into the bloodstream.

The production of ketone bodies can be triggered by various circumstances. Some of them are definitely undesirable, such as starvation and untreated type 1 diabetes, but others are positively beneficial. These include judicious fasting, intense exercise and low carbohydrate diets – all aspects of Nic's Keto Diet.

There are three main types of ketone found in the human body: beta-hydroxybutyrate (BHB), acetoacetate and acetone, the latter being a by-product of the break-down of the first two.

BHB and acetoacetate are readily extracted from the blood by cells all around the body. They are then converted into a substance called acetyl-CoA, which the cells' mitochondria use to generate energy – very efficiently.

Increasing the number of ketone bodies in the bloodstream is the immediate goal of my and other keto diets.

What is a Keto Diet?

A keto diet is one which encourages the body to go into ketosis. Provided you a) eat less fat than you are burning off to provide yourself with energy, and b) don't interfere with the process by eating more than the recommended quantities of carbohydrates and protein, you will lose body fat. You will also have much more energy than before, be less susceptible to a variety of diseases, experience great mental clarity and generally feel fantastic.

My keto diet shares some features with the Atkins Diet, notably an emphasis on drastically reducing carbohydrate intake. But its results are much more durable. It also avoids the big mistake Dr Atkins made: he failed to spot that eating large amounts of protein can lead to increased body fat, even if you eat very little carbohydrate. This happens via a process called gluconeogenesis. The word literally means 'formation of new glucose molecules'.

GLUCONEOGENESIS

Many life-forms, including animals, plants, fungi and bacteria, are able to manufacture glucose molecules from non-carbohydrate sources, including proteins and fats. This process is known as gluconeogenesis. In animals, its function is to prevent hypoglycaemia (dangerously low blood glucose).

Ruminant animals like cattle 'do' gluconeogenesis all the time. They have to, because the organisms living in their stomachs tend to grab all the carbohydrates in their food, leaving the animals needing to source glucose from elsewhere. In most other mammals, including humans, gluconeogenesis only occurs under conditions of fasting, starvation, low-carbohydrate diet or intense exercise. People in states of ketosis have low levels of blood sugar by definition. Their bodies are therefore primed for gluconeogenesis. If they eat excessive amounts of protein, this will cause body fat to accumulate.

When we eat carbohydrates, the body breaks them down into glucose molecules. In gluconeogenesis, the opposite happens. The body builds glucose molecules, using substances obtained from the breakdown of non-carbohydrate foods. In the case of protein, the relevant substances are amino acids.

The body can only utilise limited quantities of the amino acids we get from protein. Meanwhile, its ability to store them is minimal, as is the quantity we are able to excrete. So, when we eat too much protein, the excess gets sent to the liver for gluconeogenesis.

Dr Jason Fung MD, who is one of my heroes, puts it this way: "Amino acids cannot be stored for long term energy. Any protein eaten in excess needs to be converted to glucose or fat for storage". And as we know already, the body can't store very much glycogen (glucose stored as fuel).

The conclusion is clear: if we eat too much protein, we end up putting on weight in the form of body fat.

Keto and Disease

Ketogenic diets have been shown to have beneficial effects on many common diseases. Below I look at eight of the most significant. I then provide a far-from-exhaustive list of other conditions that the diet is either proven to help or strongly suspected of doing so.

Obesity

In 2016, according to the World Health Organisation, over 1.9 billion adults aged 18 or over were overweight. This equates to almost 4 in 10. Of those 1.9 billion, more than 650 million – 13% of the planet's adult population - were categorised as clinically obese (defined as having a BMI in excess of 30).

The worldwide incidence of obesity had almost tripled since 1975. The statistics were even worse for children. The percentage of five to 19-year-olds categorised as obese had multiplied more than sevenfold during the same period.

Keto diets help people lose weight in two main ways: they reduce appetite and the lowered level of insulin encourages the body to use fat rather than glucose as its primary energy source.

Diabetes

Diabetes is a disease that causes elevated levels of sugar in the blood over a prolonged period. In 2015, it was estimated that 415 million people were suffering from the condition worldwide, which equated to 8.3% of the planet's adult population.

The keto diet challenges our basic assumptions about diabetes. But before we go any further, it is essential to distinguish between type one diabetes, in which the pancreas is incapable of producing enough insulin, from the type two version of the disease. The latter, at least in its early stages, is all about insulin resistance. This is what happens when the cells of the body fail to respond properly to the hormone. They become desensitised to it, and all sorts of bad things happen as a result.

The American Diabetes Association describes type 2 diabetes as progressive and incurable. Dr Eric Westman MD, Dr Jason Fung MD and others have shown this to be incorrect (see Appendix 2). But to discover that this is the case, we have to drastically rethink the way we treat the disease. You don't give alcohol to an alcoholic to cure him. So why on earth do we give insulin to people who are addicted to it? Sure, in the short run they'll feel better. So will a 'cold-turkeying' heroin addict if you give him or her a shot of diamorphine.

Several studies have demonstrated that Type 2 diabetics who go on keto diets can find themselves able to dispense with the insulin injections they previously depended on. As they are now using fat as the primary fuel for their bodies, they no longer need to worry about high blood sugar levels caused by eating too much carbohydrate.

Heart Disease

Cardiovascular disease (CVD) is the number one killer in the world. According to the World Health Organisation, 31% of all deaths that occurred in 2015 were the result of CVD.

Of all the problems ketogenic diets can help us tackle, heart disease is probably the most important. As I stated in the introduction, my own heart was recently described as like that of a very healthy 18-year-old. But don't just take my word for it. Numerous studies have confirmed the beneficial effects keto can have on heart disease. Research published by Dr Jeff Volek and Dr Richard Feinman in 2005, for example, found that a restricted carbohydrate diet improved five key contributors to heart disease: high blood sugar, high blood triglycerides, high blood pressure and low levels of 'good' HDL cholesterol.

Epilepsy

As I mentioned on Page 41, the ketogenic diet was actually developed to treat children with drug resistant epilepsy (at the Mayo Clinic in Minnesota during the early 1920s). Numerous studies have confirmed that ketogenic diets can help with the condition. In an article published in 2013, EH Kossoff and HS Wang of the Johns Hopkins University, Baltimore state that 50-60% of epileptic children treated with keto diets will have a seizure reduction of at least 50%, while more than 1 in 10 will stop having seizures altogether.

Cancer

It is far too early to state with confidence that keto can cure certain types of cancer and much more research needs to be done. But two things are undoubtedly true. First, the use of ketogenic diets to treat cancer is rapidly growing in popularity, with many patients reporting enormous benefits. Second, many types of cancer cell can only survive by using glucose as a fuel source. It must be born in mind that cancer cells are clever, and some of the ones that rely on sugar in their early stages can learn to live on lactates and other substances.

Parkinson's Disease

Although the studies have been small, ketogenic diets have proven to be extremely helpful to people with Parkinson's disease. In 2005, five sufferers followed a keto diet for 28 days. All of them reported improved symptoms in the unified Parkinson's disease rating scale.

Autism

One of the most promising areas of keto research is the treatment of autism. The internet is filled with accounts of autistic people who have been helped by keto diets.

One study involved 30 autistic children placed on a ketogenic diet for 6 months, 30% of it made up of MCT oil. All the subjects displayed significant improvements in their condition, particularly the children on the milder end of the spectrum. Even more encouragingly, these persisted after the end of the study.

Polycystic Ovary Syndrome

Polycystic ovary syndrome causes a range of hormonal issues in woman, including infertility. It is frequently accompanied by insulin resistance, which keto diets are known to reduce.

One study, published in 2005, of eleven women with PCOS placed on a keto diet for a six-month period was so successful that two of them became pregnant during the trial!

Other Health Benefits

Keto has been shown to have beneficial effects on numerous other conditions and diseases, with degrees of certainty varying from 'very promising' to 'definite'.

I don't want to overburden you with supporting evidence at this stage – that will be provided in a future publication – but I do want to give you an idea of the potential scope of keto.

Irritable Bowel Syndrome (IBS)

Eating more fat can increase the symptoms of IBS in the short run but in the long-term a keto diet can ease them considerably. This is partly a matter of the reduced consumption of sugar, which has been shown to be good for IBS in several studies.

I used to have IBS all the time. Now it's no longer an issue.

Ageing

One way to increase lifespan is to lower oxidative stress in the body. There is good evidence that this can be done by lowering insulin levels, which ketogenic diets do.

Brain and Heart Function

The consultant cardiologist Dr Gabriela Segura has found that both the brain and the heart run at least 25% more efficiently on ketones than blood sugar.

More Energy

Mitochondria are the power stations in our cells. Dr Gabriela Segura, mentioned above, states that "the mitochondria... work much better on a ketogenic diet as they are able to increase energy levels in a stable, long-burning, efficient, and steady way... [They] are specifically designed to use fat for energy".

People on keto diets, including myself, also report less variation in energy levels.

Less Inflammation

Ketosis has been shown to have anti-inflammatory properties. This fits in with my extremely low C-Protein score mentioned in the introduction. Inflammation causes all kinds of problems in the body, so reducing it has an excellent effect on health.

Fatty Liver Disease

It stands to reason that a diet that encourages the body to burn off fat will reduce the quantity stored in the liver. I used to suffer from Fatty Liver Disease but I don't any longer. An important aspect of the PhD study I will be carrying out (see chapter 21) will be looking at the effects of my diet on this condition.

Migraines

Many migraine sufferers have reported reductions in both frequency and severity when they switched to ketogenic diets.

Heartburn/Acid Reflux

The Journal of Digestive Diseases and Sciences has reported that sufferers from acid reflux experienced a considerable reduction of symptoms when they switched to a ketogenic diet

Mood Stabilisation

I have discussed the benefits of keto diets for people with autism on Page 53. There are also numerous reports of ketosis helping people with bipolar disorders.

Alzheimer's Disease

Some scientists think Alzheimer's is really a third type of diabetes. The disease is characterised by the brain becoming less and less able to utilise glucose, causing inflammation and other problems.

We know that the brain can power itself very efficiently with ketones. There are therefore good reasons to expect keto diets to be helpful for the condition, and an increasing number of studies are offering support for this theory.

Multiple Sclerosis (MS)

At this stage the evidence is mostly anecdotal, but studies with mice suggest that ketogenic diets may be very helpful for people with MS.

Acne

There is increasing evidence that keto diets are good for acne-reduction. We know that foods that yield lots of glucose can cause outbreaks of acne, so it makes sense that a diet that eliminates them would have a beneficial effect on the condition.

Who Should NOT do a Keto Diet

The keto diet is wonderful and transformative, but it isn't for everybody. If you have type 1 diabetes, for instance, doing it would be very risky indeed.

If you are in any doubt about whether my diet is safe for you given your medical profile, please consult your doctor. Actually, do this anyway. Apart from anything else, it is essential that doctors get to see what keto can do for their clients' health first-hand.

There is a fairly full but not exhaustive list of conditions which are not compatible with doing my diet in Appendix 1 at the end of this book. PLEASE READ THIS BEFORE YOU GO ANY FURTHER.

I am sometimes asked whether my diet would pose a risk to people with a history of eating disorders. Leaving aside the fact that a high-fat diet is unlikely to appeal to someone with anorexia, for example, my answer is that eating disorders are primarily psychological (though they obviously have physical effects), whereas my diet is primarily physical (though it has psychological effects). It will not, therefore, address the root cause of eating disorders.

Keto and Children

Lots of my friends on keto say "I wouldn't let my children do it". Why not, provided their doctors are OK with it? Give them their vitamins and a little bit of fruit and they'll be more than fine. They will also not be learning dietary habits and developing insulin resistance that would plague them throughout their lives.

We have been systematically taught that eating fruit is essential, particularly for children. In fact, fructose, the dominant sugar in fruit, is even worse than regular sugar from an obesity perspective. It doesn't get converted into muscle glycogen. Instead, once you exceed the very small quantity that can be stored in the liver, it is turned straight into body fat. There is nowhere else for it to go.

Milk is better, as it contains only about 4% sugar (in the form of lactose), as opposed to 40-50% for some fruit juices. But it still isn't ideal, except for babies.

The FDA has recently taken out the recommendation that thirsty kids should be given fruit juice to drink. It now advocates water instead. This is a very good thing. Apple juice contains more sugar than Coke!

The British TV chef Jamie Oliver did a study of commercial baby food and found that most of it was stuffed with carrot and apple. This teaches infants to rely on sugar as an energy source.

3

PART THREE – NIC'S KETO DIET

Why do my Diet? – The Benefits

My wife says "if I don't eat sugar and fruit, I won't be happy". Well, I'm not suggesting you do my diet to be virtuous. I'm suggesting you do it precisely to make yourself happy.

My diet can't solve every problem in your life – some damage from the past cannot be undone – but If you have previously had an unhealthy lifestyle, it can certainly help you have a better future. I like to look at it this way. Imagine you were born with $100 deposited in a bank account. On average, this should buy you 100 years. If you spend $60 in your first 40 years, you can cut down your expenditure to make your remaining $40 last for 60.

I have listed several of the specific diseases keto diets are known to help on page 49-56. The more general benefits include the following:

Weight Loss

This is obviously the prime motivation for most people to take up my diet.

Sometimes, when I'm at the gym, I pick up a weight corresponding to the amount of fat I have shed (40kg/88lb) to remind myself what it was like carrying around that extra burden. I can scarcely walk with it.

Mental Clarity

Weight loss aside, for me the best thing about being on the keto diet is the mental clarity it brings. Mine is a fast-mimicking diet, which means that it gives you the benefits associated with fasting without you actually doing it. When I am in ketosis, I sometimes feel I have access to what I call the fourth dimension, a state in which I have an overview of everything that is going on that is qualitatively different from anything else I have experienced. I don't particularly advocate trying to achieve high ketone scores – for my diet to work, all that matters is that you go into ketosis – but if you do get into that zone, in my experience it's like flying on a cloud. Your head is so clear and your body so light that you feel you can travel across time.

I have always been struck by how many of the philosophers and great religious thinkers went in for fasting, including Christian Monks and Hindu and Buddhist teachers. When politicians assemble to make major decisions, I think it would be a very good idea for them to be on keto diets! Maybe the hunger that comes first would make some of them more compassionate, while the follow-up ketosis could make them more visionary.

One thing needs to be born in mind though. To get fat, you need time. To ruin your mental clarity, one ill-advised meal is enough.

Mental Health

Losing weight definitely has a beneficial effect on the mental wellbeing of those who were previously obese. It stands to reason that people are going to feel better about themselves if they make improvements to a condition that is so obviously detrimental to their health.

When I was big, I used to worry constantly that I had cancer. If you're fat, you suffer from all sorts of aches and pains, and these provide food for the worrying machine. And if your head is sick, you tend to eat more. It's a vicious circle.

More research needs to be done, but it seems very likely that keto has a beneficial effect on depression and helps to prevent it occurring. This is certainly my experience. Fasting for extended periods is different. If you don't think positively while you are doing it, you can get depressed as the experience of not eating can create anxiety, which will feed negative thoughts if you are not careful.

Sexual Performance

One of the biggest bonuses of the keto diet is its effect on your sexual performance. Let's face it, nobody minds functioning better in that department. If you fast for a week, you probably will have a problem with your libido but the opposite is true with intermittent fasting. I don't want to give too much away here, but in my direct experience, it can turn a three-minute man into a 20 minute one.

Looking Good

Everyone feels happy when they know they look good. If you follow my keto diet, this is pretty much guaranteed. People who have known me a long time sometimes beg me to tell them the secret of the transformation of my appearance.

Time

Another benefit of my diet is the amount of time it saves you. Shopping and cooking become much simpler. For Americans in particular, this is very good news, as they tend to equate time with money!

Money

While I'm on that subject, many people worry that going on my diet will be expensive, because of its insistence on organic products, grass-fed meat and so on. It is true that you will be paying more for what you buy than you would for the non-organic, factory farmed equivalents. But you will be saving a great deal of money by not buying all sorts of things that your body doesn't need. On balance, you are likely to be better off than before.

Freedom

You have the right to be free and the first part of your freedom is not to be dependent on anything harmful outside yourself. Sugar definitely falls into that category.

In my understanding, human beings as God created them are free. They were not constrained by anything either external or internal until they sinned, as described in powerful poetic language in the 'Garden of Eden' story. But once they had done this, they became slaves to greed and obsessed with power, sex and food.

As history and technology have progressed, people have become increasingly freed from the bondage imposed by external factors like poverty and disease. But we can only enjoy the reality of our freedom if we are not bound by obsessions, worries and addictions. Our societies pay a great deal of attention to some of the most obviously addictive substances, like tobacco, alcohol and narcotics, but they tend to overlook what may be the most harmful one of all. This is the hidden killer present in most of our food and drinks: SUGAR.

How My Diet is Different

Nic's Keto Diet (NKD) was developed in the light of a growing trend for keto dieting, for which there is now a multi-billion-dollar market in the United States alone. It is a simplified version of the original keto diet that still produces incredible results. It involves a combination of intermittent fasting, mindful eating and an emphasis on organic products.

The key features which distinguish my approach from other keto diets are:

- Its simplification of the process
- The integration of intermittent fasting and exercise
- The integration of mindful eating
- Much more emphasis on greens and vegetables (inspired by Dr. Eric Berg DC, another inspirational keto and intermittent fasting speaker). Aside from keeping you healthy and adding variety, these foods help prevent constipation, which is often a problem with the Atkins and other low carb diets

MINDFUL EATING

Mindfulness – focusing the attention on the present moment - is all the rage nowadays. It can be applied as much to eating and drinking as to anything else.

Mindful eating involves:

• Eating slowly, without distraction.

• Paying close attention to the sensory qualities of your food: colour, aroma, taste, mouthfeel and texture. This makes eating a much more satisfying experience.

• Learning to distinguish between genuine hunger and 'conditioned' triggers for eating (e.g. "It's 1pm so I must be hungry").

• Stopping eating when you are full.

• Learning to deal with anxiety and guilt about food.

• Being aware of the effects different foods have on your feelings and well-being.

Intermittent Fasting

Intermittent Fasting (IF) is an important element of my diet. It's not compulsory but it is hugely beneficial.

Before I go any further, DO NOT GET INTO A PANIC ABOUT THE WORD 'FASTING'! I'm not suggesting that you ever go as much as a full day without eating. It's just a matter of learning to leave a long period between your last meal of the day and your first meal of the next one. Once you are in ketosis, this will be easy, as you won't experience hunger pangs. The fact that you are fasting will also make it much easier for you to go into and stay in ketosis. It's a virtuous circle.

In a nutshell, intermittent fasting (IF) is all about lengthening the proportion of the day when you don't eat anything at all. I didn't do it on purpose in the beginning. It happened naturally because I didn't feel hungry. But then I did some research – Dr Jason Fung MD was a major inspiration - and found that the benefits were enormous. Above all, IF helps you achieve ketosis much faster than you otherwise would. And, because you are relying less on the food you have eaten, particularly towards the end of the fasting period, IF encourages your system to start using body fat as a fuel. The result is faster weight loss.

Some people advocate eating only one meal per day but I prefer to eat two. Initially, I left 12 hours between them but now the gap is down to four. I realise, however, that this won't appeal to everybody. So I recommend the 16/8 method as a good starting point. This involves splitting your day into a 16-hour period of fasting and an 8 hour eating window. You could, for instance, have your first meal of the day at 11am and your second at 7pm. An 18/6 ratio would be even better.

People tend to get very nervous when confronted with the idea of not eating for a period. "But you'll die!" they say, "or at least become weak and unhealthy". In fact, the opposite is true, at least for the kind of fasting I'm advocating, which is for very short periods.

If you're in any doubt about this, consider the case of Angus Barbieri. During 1965 and 1966, this 27-year-old Scotsman went 382 days without eating any food at all, although he did take vitamin supplements. He did it under the supervision of the University Department of Medicine at the Royal Infirmary of Dundee. The doctors there initially advised him to fast for just a few days but when he decided to prolong the process, they supported him and said they'd keep an eye on him. His weight fell from 207kg/456lbs to 82kg/180lbs and he stayed healthy throughout. His system was able to find all the resources it needed from his stores of body fat.

Our ancestors often hadn't eaten for a couple of days. In that condition, they needed to be even better at hunting than usual. So, our systems are actually designed to give us more energy when we haven't eaten for a period.

Some of the politicians reading this will have inadvertently experienced the mental benefits of fasting when stuck in their debating chambers for extended periods. The fact is, you get sharper if you abstain from eating when you normally would have, at least in the short run.

Paradoxically, intermittent fasting helps you to avoid hunger pangs. This is connected to a hormone called ghrelin, which is produced by the stomach to stimulate appetite. The levels of ghrelin in the blood rise just before we are accustomed to eating. If we fast, this continues to happen for about three days, but then the ghrelin spikes stop. For this reason, people who are fasting tend to stop feeling hungry after three or four days. The same is true of people who fast intermittently, although the effect is less pronounced and takes a bit longer to kick in.

Exercise

Like intermittent fasting, exercise is a very desirable aspect of my diet but not absolutely essential. Don't think I'm going to let you off the hook though!

The great virtue of exercise for people on a keto diet is that it speeds up the rate at which you burn body fat. When I've finished a session at the gym, I go on a machine that measures this. It also gives a 'metabolic age'. In 18 months, mine has gone down from 56 to 32.

I never did any exercise when I was young. I always skipped it. Now, my gym in London is my second office. I'm a religious man, so I'm not out to hook women, but I can't deny I love it when a female half my age glances at me appreciatively through the side of her eyes while I'm in the gym. It's another star in my book.

If you really can't face going to the gym, the good news is that the extra energy and weight loss that keto brings will make you want to move around more than you used to anyway.

One thing you should be aware of is that exercise builds muscle. This will slow down your weight loss, but the goal of my diet is

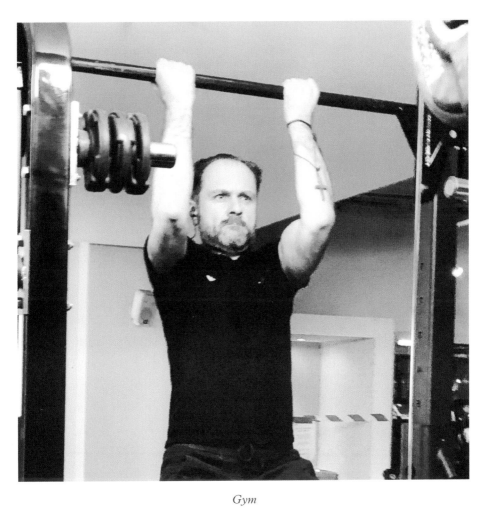

Gym

improved health and reduced body fat, not weight loss per se. Reshaping your body is the priority and it's also the most difficult thing to do. Measure the body fat on your belly and thighs from time to time. If this is reducing, don't get depressed, even if your weight is stagnant. Things are moving in the right direction!

Almost needless to say, steroids are very bad for keto. People who are using the for medical reasons rather than body building often find that the diet renders them unnecessary, or at least reduces the need for them.

A final tip: to get the most benefit from your exercises, try to do them while in a fasted state. This is always my aim.

Macros

'Macros' is short for 'macronutrients'. The word refers to the three categories of food that provide us with calories: protein, fat and carbohydrate. If we want to lose weight, we need to establish how much of each we should be eating per day. The desirable quantities will depend on several individual factors, including age, height, weight, activity levels and how much weight you want to lose.

To work out the amount of each food group you should be eating, you need to use a 'macro calculator.

The general macros for Nic's Keto Diet are 75% Fat, 20% Protein, 5% Carbs (not more than 20g a day). But you need to do the calculations because the optimum ratios can vary between individuals.

Keto Flu and Other Concerns

Keto Flu and How to Avoid it

Although the keto diet is easy once your body has adjusted, you can definitely feel off-colour at times during the first few days. This is because your body, which has been used to powering itself by burning sugar, is transitioning to a new fuel – fat. It knows exactly how to do this but it does take it a little while to adapt. This is even more true of your mind.

While the adaption is taking place, you may suffer from various flu-like symptoms such as headaches, tiredness, dizziness or irritability. You are withdrawing from a powerful drug, which you have been using for your entire life, so it's not surprising that your body and mind protest a bit at first.

Some people give up at this stage. They remind me of a friend of mine who went swimming in the ocean in Brazil. I asked him if he'd enjoyed it and he said he hadn't, because he couldn't get out of the shallows and into the deep water. Every time he tried, a big wave knocked him over.

Fortunately, there are lots of techniques to help you through the waves. Drinking a lot of water and adding electrolytes helps, because as I explained on page 80, you pee a lot in the initial stages of the keto diet. This is due to the body using up its glycogen reserves, which are tied up with water molecules. But the real secret is MCT oil, which is usually derived from coconut oil. The initials stand for 'Medium Chain Triglycerides'.

To cut a long story short, the body finds it very easy to convert MCT oil into fuel for ketosis. Inside the body, it skips most of the usual digestive processes and is diverted directly from the small intestine to the liver, where it is broken down into ketones.

If you consume small amounts of MCT oil, perhaps mixed in with your coffee, you will start going into ketosis much sooner tha you otherwise would. It only takes an hour or so for the process to start, whereas it can take several days for your body to switch from burning carbohydrate to fat. The MCT oil kick-starts the transition, providing almost instant energy and banishing most of the symptoms of keto flu.

To return to the wave analogy, once you are in the deep water, you are very hard to tempt because you feel full.

N.B. If you take MCTs while you're still eating enough carbohydrates to supply your body's energy needs, your body will store them as fat. MCTs won't make you slim on their own.

Muscle

A concern some people have about keto is that it will cause them to lose muscle. You do lose a tiny amount at first but not once you are fat-adapted. When your body burns protein, the level of urea in your blood rises sharply. Studies of individuals who are fasting have shown that they do not have elevated levels of urea, which implies that they are not using up muscle. They would if they had literally no body fat, but this isn't something most people need worry about, particularly those embarking on diets!

My diet places more emphasis on the conservation of muscle than many other versions of keto.

Cholesterol

As I explained in Chapter 6, the idea that cholesterol is the root of all evil has been etched deeply into our minds, largely because of some badly flawed science. There is no getting around the fact that my keto diet is high in cholesterol. But as many studies have shown, notable the Feldman Protocol), the more cholesterol you eat, the less of it you tend to have in your bloodstream. This may seem bizarre but it's similar to the fundamental principle behind the keto diet: if you eat a lot of fat as a ratio of your total food consumption, you'll store less of it in your body.

What to Eat, How Much and When

As with all diets, the key to success with my version is to eat fewer calories than you burn up. But the great thing about ketosis is that once you are in it, you don't feel hungry. This makes this diet much easier than many others. Still, without discipline, nothing works.

First I'll give you some general principles, then I'll provide some specific lists.

Millennials are often described as the 'avocado and toast'

generation. My diet is **'avocado and eggs, plus butter'**. Avocados are great. They contain 'good' carbohydrates that don't spike your insulin. And eggs are hugely important to my eating regime. I eat about six a day, always making sure they come from grass-fed chickens, or at least free-range birds. Hard boiled ones are best, because they fill you up more.

In England, where I spend much of my time, two of the national staples are bread and butter, and fish and chips. If you tweak that to **'fish and butter'**, with a side order of greens, you have the essence of my diet in a nutshell.

Keto is often described as **'the bacon diet'**. This is an appealing idea for most people – I even know lifelong

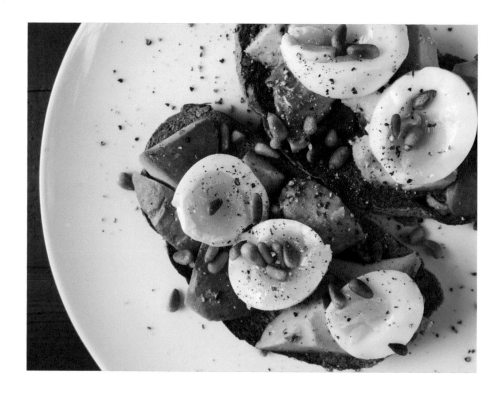

vegetarians who are entranced by the smell of cooking bacon – but it's only true up to a point. In some ways, it's an ideal keto food, as it consists of a little bit of protein and lots of fat, but it also usually contains nitrates, which are harmful. Obviously, you should avoid the sweet-cured kind. You should also be aware of the possibility of other types of meat being 'tainted' with sugar. It is often an ingredient in the rubs applied to barbecued items, for example.

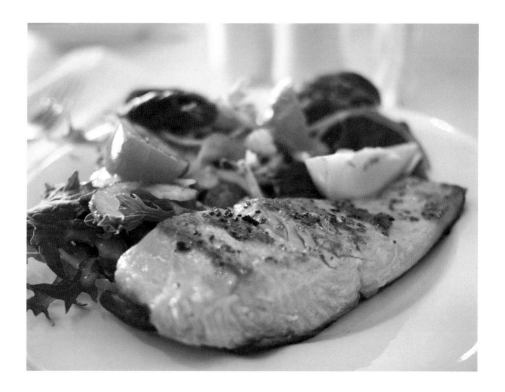

FOOD LABELLING

Food labelling is notorious for its potential to mislead, and you need to be very careful about it. Supermarkets and manufacturers go out of their way to give us more favourable impressions of their products than their reality deserves.

The term 'grass-fed' is a case in point. All it means is that the animal that provided the meat will have been fed grass for some portion of its life. It may well have spent its last few months being fattened on a wholly or partially grain-based diet. To add to the confusion, 'grass-fed' doesn't necessarily mean 'raised on pasture'. The phrase you should look for on the label is 'grass-finished'. This means that the animal ate nothing but grass and forage for its entire life. Grass-finished beef is 20% lower in calories than the grain-finished equivalent and has higher levels of Omega-3 fatty acids, CLA (Conjugated Linoleic Acid — an essential fatty acid that fights cancer and inhibits body fat), and Vitamins A and E. You also need to be very wary of the practice of calling sugars and starches by names that most people wouldn't recognise as such. Monosodium Glutamate (MSG), for example, is often added to foods to make them more palatable and more-ish. It is bad news if you are on my diet anyway, as it makes you want to eat more, but the worst thing about it is that it takes you out of ketosis.

Manufacturers know that health conscious people will avoid buying anything labelled as containing MSG, so they use terms like 'modified starch' 'maltodextrin' or 'hydrolysed protein' instead.

Another thing to avoid is 'whey isolate', which shoots your insulin up immediately. And there are a bewildering number of disguised names for sugar, ranging from dextrin to evaporated cane juice and xylose.

- **Oils** are vital to my diet. Separated fats like tallow and ghee are excellent for frying, although you mustn't let the temperature get too high or they start to alter chemically. The best vegetable oils for my diet are avocado, coconut, olive and MCT. Use them liberally to dress salads.

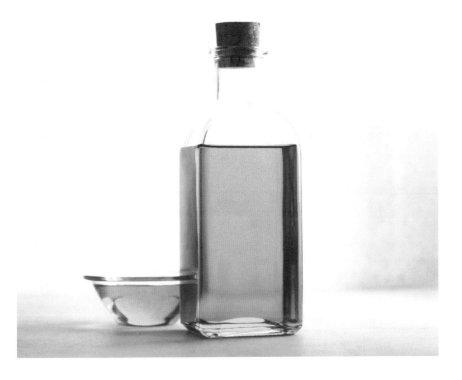

• **Fermented foods** like sauerkraut and kimchee are essential to keeping your gut bacteria in balance. You need to make sure you buy (or make) unsweetened versions though. I eat around 50g/2oz per day, but some of my Russian friends eat 0.5kg/1lb in a sitting!

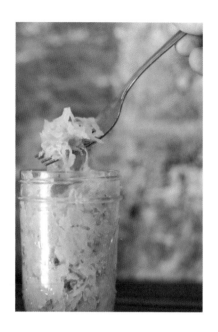

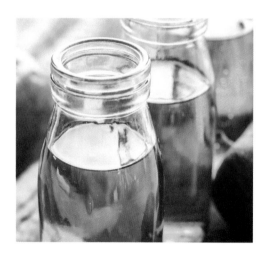

• **Apple cider vinegar** is another great product. It helps clean your system. There is more information about it in the appendix section on essentials.

It is very important to stick to organic food when on my diet. In fact, my trademark is 'Nic's Keto and Organic'. As I've said before, it is too simplistic to say "you are what you eat", but it's definitely true that if you eat an animal product, you end up consuming some of what the animal consumed. Leaving aside ethical considerations, the biggest problem with non-organic food is the effect it can have on hormone regulation.

WHERE TO BUY YOUR FOOD

To do Nic's Keto Diet properly, you need to source good, organic food free of nasty additives.

Personally, I buy most of my groceries from Whole Foods Market. I don't have any financial interest in the company but I have to admit I'm addicted to the place. This excellent organic supermarket chain has almost 500 outlets in the USA and United Kingdom. Meanwhile, lots of organic shops are opening all around Europe, which is a very promising tendency.

Whole Foods do sell sugary treats, but they also have everything you need for my diet. It's guaranteed to be free of harmful, non-natural additives, genetically modified ingredients, meat injected with growth hormones and so on.

It isn't the cheapest place to shop but as I've said elsewhere, you'll be saving a great deal of money by cutting out all the carb-heavy things excluded by my diet.

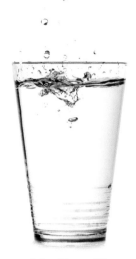

You need to drink plenty of water on my diet, because when fat cells are destroyed they release toxins which need to be flushed out of your system. You should also make sure there is some salt in your diet, to compensate for that lost through urination. Some dieters are tempted to ignore the water advice to get a slightly better result when they stand on their scales, but I strongly discourage this.

My diet will provide you with all the nutrients you need, but it's not a bad idea to take some supplements, particularly magnesium and vitamin D. The reason for the first is that keto makes you wee more than you used to, so you lose magnesium through urination. The second is advisable because almost nobody gets as much sunlight as is needed for the body to manufacture what it requires.

Weighing yourself is very important. Personally, I do it several times a day, because I am micro-interested in the fluctuations and their causes, but you don't need to do this. What you do need is a good set of scales and to weigh yourself at the same time every day. The best time to do this is in the morning, after you've been to the bathroom but before you drink anything.

I am sometimes asked whether my diet is suitable for doing on and off; 'on' when you want or need to lose weight, 'off' when you don't. My answer is that is perfectly possible, but it's not what I'm advocating. I'm recommending a complete change in lifestyle. Once you've experienced the benefits, why would you want to go back to the old way?

One last thing to bear in mind. In the early stages of my diet, you will probably lose weight even if you exceed the recommended quantities of food, provided you stick to the ratios. This is because your hormones will be better regulated. This won't be enough in the long run but it's nice while it lasts.

So, let's get down to the specifics!

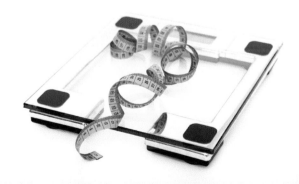

Daily Recommendations

<u>Greens/Vegetables</u>

200 to 300g/7-10 oz, made up from any of the following:

Lettuce (all kinds are good)
Rucola/rocket
Spinach (better raw)
Mushrooms
Asparagus
A little bit of broccoli

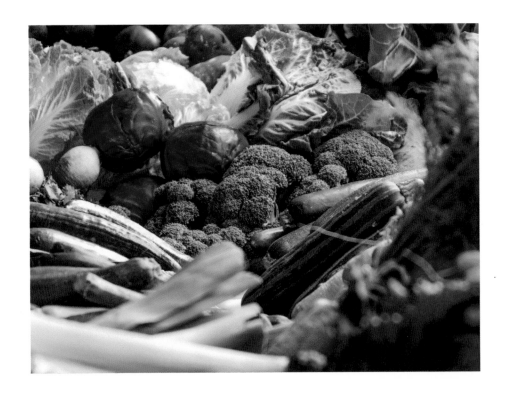

Fats and Oils

Organic and grass-fed sources are always best. The following are all good:

Fatty fish
Animal fat (non-hydrogenated)
Lard
Tallow
Butter from grass-fed animals
Avocados
Egg yolks
Macadamia/brazil nuts
Butter/ghee
Mayonnaise
Coconut gutter
Cocoa gutter
Olive oil
Coconut oil
Avocado oil
Macadamia oil
MCT oil

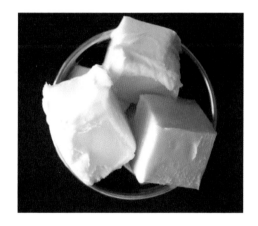

I find the three most valuable items on this list are MCT oil, olive oil and grass-fed butter. They are sufficient on their own to provide all the fats you need.

<u>Protein</u>

Again, organic and grass-fed sources are always to be preferred.

Fish - Preferably eating anything that is caught wild, such as catfish, cod, flounder, halibut, mackerel, mahi-mahi, salmon, snapper, trout, and tuna. Fattier fish is better.

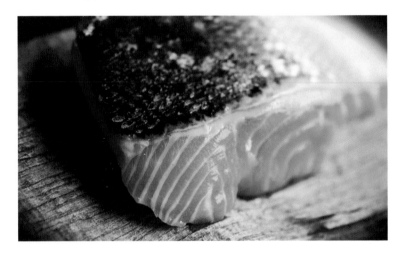

Shellfish - Clams, oysters, lobster, crab, scallops, mussels, and squid.

Whole Eggs - Try to get them free-range from the local market if possible. You can prepare them in many different ways: fried, devilled, boiled, poached, scrambled and so on.

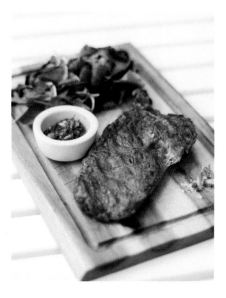

Beef - Ground beef, steak, roasts, and stew meat. Stick with fattier cuts where possible.

Pork - Ground pork, pork loin, pork chops, tenderloin, and ham. Watch out for added sugars and try to stick with fattier cuts.

Poultry - Chicken, duck, quail, pheasant and other wild game.

Offal/Organ - Heart, liver, kidney, and tongue. Offal is one of the best sources of vitamins/nutrients.

Other Meat - Veal, goat, lamb, turkey and all kinds of wild game not previously mentioned. Stick with fattier cuts where possible.

Bacon and Sausage - Check labels and avoid anything cured in sugar or containing artificial fillers. Don't be overly concerned about nitrates but you're better off without them.

What to Avoid

• Imbalance of Omega 6 and Omega 3 fats. Omega 3 is the 'good' one, being a vital component of cell membranes and important in the manufacture of hormones. Omega 6 is less good. You do need some of it but too much of it causes inflammation. Ideally, when you are on my diet, the ratio of six to three should be about one to one. In the typical American diet, it is more like 15 to one.

• All sweeteners other than erythritol and pure stevia. Monk fruit has a noticeable effect on the taste of food.

• Soya or other hormone stimulating ingredients (even though they are considered healthy). Soya is a big no-no. Yes, it's high in protein and low in carbohydrate, but it contains compounds which are very similar to human oestrogen. Too much of it can cause men to develop 'man boobs'. Tofu should be excellent on the basis of its macro profile, but its hormonal effects rule it out for my diet.

• Grains - They contain far more carbohydrate than our bodies evolved to expect. How are cows fattened ahead of slaughter? They are fed grain.

• Peas and pulses - These are not a good idea either. They have too much sugar in them and you don't need them, as you'll be getting plenty of protein from elsewhere.

• Excessive quantities of calcium - You do need some of it in your diet – it's essential for strong teeth and bones - but in my opinion pro-calcium propaganda has gone way too far.

Too much calcium can lead to a build-up of plaque in your arteries. I don't take it as a supplement and my bones are 4% denser than they used to be as a result of me doing weights at the gym.

• Non-fat snacking, to prevent periodic spikes of insulin.

• Protein bars, shakes and supplements, which are often full of sugar and/or insulin spiking sweeteners. Even when they are not, excessive protein consumption will take you out of ketosis via the process of gluconeogenesis (see page 47)

• Avoid picking unnecessary fights and don't flirt with food. It can't say "no" to you. If you do put yourself in tempting situations, you'll become stressed, which will raise your levels of the 'flight or fight' hormone cortisol. When this happens, keto doesn't work properly, because the message the body gets is "you are in danger. Retain your fat in case you need it".

• Don't eat while you are watching TV because it makes it hard to monitor what you are doing.

• Never eat just because of habit or a sense of duty. We have cheated the hormones that make us feel hungry or full (ghrelin and leptin respectively) by overriding their messages and confusing them with sugar. We need to learn to listen to them again.

Getting Started

Dealing with Resistance

When you tell people what you are planning to do, not everybody is going to give you a big pat on the back. You can expect resistance of two kinds: first, from those who are ignorant of the science, but wedded to the old 'fat is bad' belief; second, from people who are scared that they might have to change their lifestyles if what you say is true and they don't attack it.

You are particularly likely to face opposition from two groups of people: the medical profession, and family and friends.

Resistance from the Medical Profession

My sister is on the diet and losing weight. Her husband, who is a surgeon, initially said "what is your brother trying to do to you?", despite himself having tried several 'conventional' diets without success. Then she showed him some pro-keto scientific material on the internet and he said "OK, maybe there's something in it after all".

At the time of writing, there is only one respected university course about the keto diet out there, at Duke University in North Carolina. This needs to change. From my perspective as someone heavily involved in the training of doctors, the problem is simple. When it comes to nutritional information, nearly all of them have drunk from the same contaminated well: the flawed science taught in med schools.

If, as I strongly advise, you go to see your doctor before starting my diet, you can expect some resistance, because it goes against everything they are likely to have been taught ('fat is the enemy'). I therefore suggest you don't ask "do you think this is a good idea?" Instead, say "I want to do this, so please help me". If they refuse, ask them to explain why and be prepared to argue the case for keto. If they say "I don't want to hear about it", alarm bells should start ringing.

In my experience, doctors vary considerably in the extent to which they are prepared to take the claims made for keto seriously. They remind me of the different kinds of ground in the parable of the sower. Sometimes the seed lands on hard ground and has no chance of germinating. In other cases, the idea takes root.

To the sceptics I would say "remember that at one stage doctors didn't believe in germs and microbes, yet people still died from them. Remember, too, that the Catholic Church threatened to burn Galileo because he said that the Earth moved around the Sun".

Resistance from Family and Friends

My Russian mother-in-law, who lived through the Second World War, finds it particularly difficult to get her head around keto. She talks about the desperate searches for food, and the delight she would feel if she found just one small potato. But I try to clarify things to her "Eat one potato and you're full. Eat two and you're very full. But eat three and you're hungry again, because your insulin rises, telling you to eat more food. Then you'll be eating five, six or seven".

The best advice I can give you about how to get your family and friends onside is this: educate them, without being preachy. Say "I really want to try this diet, because I've heard fantastic things about it". Show them a copy of this book and direct them to some of the articles and videos listed in Appendix 2.

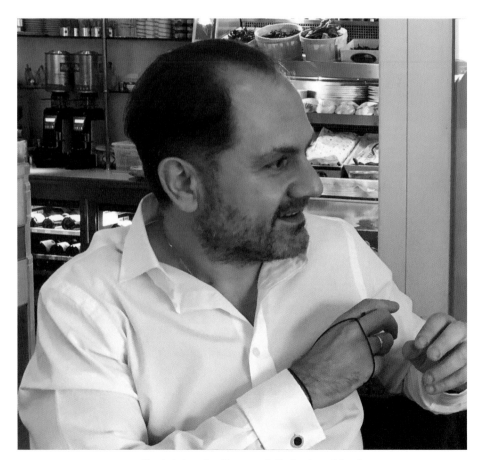

Explaining the diet on a daily basis to friends

Preparation for the Diet

DON'T STRESS!

The first thing to emphasise is this: DO NOT GET STRESSED! Aside from being unpleasant, stress raises the level of cortisol in your body, which makes it virtually impossible to lose fat. There is a good evolutionary reason for this. When our ancestors experienced the stress of being unable to find food, their endocrine systems instructed their bodies to store fat rather than burn it as they were likely to need to draw on their reserves later.

If you do find yourself getting stressed, don't compound the problem by stressing about it. Just accept that you are temporarily feeling uncomfortable. The stress will soon subside. Meanwhile, live in the moment and look forward to the joy you will experience when, in a week or a month's time, people notice how much slimmer, healthier and more active you have become.

The day before you start the diet, clean out your pantry and your fridge. The less you are confronted with all sorts of tempting things you shouldn't be eating the better. I have my own fridge at home. Not everybody has this luxury, but at least try to arrange to have your own shelf in your shared one. Then instruct your eyes not to look above or below it!

Make sure you have the following:

- A good set of scales
- A keto measuring device (see page 121). These are getting cheaper all the time.
- MCT oil
- An App to work out your macros (see pages 23 and 70)
- Enough keto-friendly food to last you for three or four days. It's not a bad idea to avoid supermarkets during this period in case you should feel tempted to buy something 'naughty'.

The First Few Days

I would recommend starting the diet on a Monday, because the chances are you'll be busy. This will help you not to obsess about food.

On the Saturday, feel free to have a blow-out, eating all the carbs you want. Personally, I'd go out to a good restaurant.

Sunday is a halfway day. Eat light and have your last meal of the day at about 5 or 6pm. In the evening, make a big batch of soup. Bone broth would be ideal. Try making it out of grass-fed, organic oxtail. Before you go to bed, tell yourself "tomorrow, I will delay my first meal of the day for as long as I can".

On the Monday, you need to follow through on this decision. Try not to eat before about 11am. Earlier in the morning, have a few sips of MCT oil (or coconut oil if you can't get hold of any) to kick-start the ketosis process and ward off keto flu. Aim to eat your evening meal no later than 8pm and preferably an hour or two earlier.

The following day repeat this pattern, then keep on going! If you don't cheat, after a week to ten days I guarantee you'll feel the difference.

As time goes on, try to push your meal times closer together until you get into a 16/8 rhythm (see page 66). Once you are in ketosis, you may experience psychological hunger but you are unlikely to feel the physical kind, so long as you follow my instructions.

A Week or so in - has the Diet Stopped Working?

Each gram of glycogen in your body is bound up with 3-4 grams of water. When your body burns up its glycogen stores, which it will do quickly when you start my diet, this water is released. As a result, you go to the bathroom a lot and lose weight very quickly. In the early stage of my diet, people typically lose around 2kg/4.4lbs in a few days. This is very gratifying but most of it is water. You won't go on getting the 'burn one gram, lose three or four for free' result for long. And as soon as you start eating carbohydrates again, you will put the 2kg on again very rapidly. This has led some people to conclude, wrongly, that the diet doesn't work. It does, but only so long as you stick to it.

If you fast, you will use up the glycogen stored in your

liver in 18 to 24 hours, faster if you exercise. In theory, at this stage you should start burning fat, but if your system isn't fat-adapted, it'll go for the glycogen in your muscles first. You have to teach it to run on fat. This takes time, as you've been teaching it to run on carbohydrates for a lifetime. Once you are fat-adapted, your body won't start drawing on the reserves of glycogen in your muscles the moment there isn't much glucose in your blood-stream.

Maintaining the Diet - Keto as a Lifestyle

A few weeks of my diet will make you lose weight but to reap the full benefits, you need to integrate it into your life. This chapter shows you some of the ways to do this

Weighing Yourself

Some experts advise people on keto diets to weigh themselves once a week. Personally, I do it ten times a day. I realise I'm unusually interested in what goes on in my body but I want to know exactly what's happening and why. Although I know that my weight will fluctuate during the day, the advantage of weighing myself so often is that it allows me to pick up on trends early.

Keeping Records/Apps

Another thing I do 'religiously' is record everything I eat and drink. And I mean everything. I heartily recommend you do the same. In fact, it's essential. It makes mistakes very easy to spot, particularly when you cross reference what you eat with what you weigh. Even a simple thing like putting too much parmesan on your salad or eating too many nuts can throw your diet out of keto temporarily. I use an App called 'Fat Secrets'. It takes me about 15 minutes but it's worth it.

Some Apps are too simplistic about fibre, which is an important part of my greens-heavy version of the keto diet. You need to distinguish between soluble fibre, which is a source of sugar, and insoluble fibre, which isn't. Other Apps are much too tolerant of sweeteners such as Maltitol, which ends up giving you at least half as many calories as sucrose, along with an insulin spike.

CALORIE COUNTING - TOTAL CARBS OR NET CARBS?

Calorie counting is not as important at the beginning of my diet as it is later – you'll lose weight regardless if you do your macros and follow my guidelines for what to eat every day - but eventually it becomes essential. This is particularly true if you go against my advice and snack during the day, because this will keep your insulin high unless you are very careful.

One thing you need to be very clear about when working out your calorie consumption is whether you are going to count total carbs or net carbs. The net figure is obtained by subtracting the fibre content from the total figure.

The problem with using the net carb approach is that the body handles soluble and insoluble fibres differently. Soluble fibres end up being converted into sugar.

Food retailers in many parts of the world are required by law to list total the carbohydrate content of their products, but many of them also do a net carb calculation, by subtracting all the fibre they contain. As we know, businesses that make their money from food often mislead, so it isn't always wise to trust their calculations.

My advice is to count total carbs.

Many experts recommend people on keto diets to consume a maximum of 35g of total carbs and 25g of net carbs per day. My own recommendation is a maximum of 20g total carbs. This will ensure you go into ketosis much more easily.

Social Life

I often get asked how doing keto affects one's social life. My answer is that socialising isn't just a matter of eating and drinking alcohol. It's about talking and communicating too. What you lose in the first area you'll more than make up for in the second. On keto, I find I talk more. I'm also far more energetic. When you are clearer in your head, you are much more interesting to other people, and vice-versa.

I also don't want to give you the impression that you can't go out to restaurants when you're on my diet. You most certainly can – you just have to be careful about what you eat and not feel shy about leaving things that are contrary to the diet on your plate. I often order a steak with a pat of butter, which keeps me very happy. Spinach is often available too.

Alcohol

Yes, you can drink a bit of alcohol without violating the principles of keto, provided it's a spirit like whisky, which has relatively little available sugar. But aside from the difficulty many people have stopping at one or two shots, the problem with alcohol is that one of its by-products is so toxic that the liver shuts down its other activities to deal with it. This stops it processing fat. If you drink while you're on my diet, you may be in ketosis sometimes but you're unlikely to lose weight.

I'd be lying if I said alcohol isn't sometimes a temptation when you're with people who are drinking it. Occasionally I do have a drink. In general, though, I avoid it. I don't really believe people who say they drink because it makes them happy, because in my experience, if you're drunk you don't know whether you're happy or sad. For me, my body is just a vehicle for my spirit. It can't function in an unhealthy vehicle with a blocked CPU (the brain).

Personally, I'm happy when I feel smart, and I'm smarter without alcohol.

When Hunger Strikes Unexpectedly

If you are doing the diet properly, in theory you won't be tempted to eat. But when I'm in low ketosis, I do find that this sometimes happens, because my leptin is relatively low and my adrenaline high. My solution is to have a slug of MCT oil in a cup of coffee before I go out. It makes all the difference. Hardboiled eggs are also good in an emergency.

Even without the MCT oil, coffee and tea, particularly the green variety, are your friends when you are doing this diet. They help you to prevent hunger pangs and they give you something sociable to do in company.

Keto and Other Popular Diets

I constantly talk to people who are trying to lose weight, and have noticed that many of them don't do pure versions of any particular diet. Instead, they mix principles from different ones.

There can be several reasons for this. Someone may have had a degree of success with a diet but discovered that they need to tweak it to make it really work for them. Or there may be some aspect of a diet that would otherwise suit them perfectly that goes contrary to their beliefs, or that they simply don't like. A person who hates brassicas is going to have a tough time with the cabbage soup diet!

In many ways, the 'tailor-made' approach is a good thing. One size does not fit all and different combinations appeal to different people. But it is important to know what mixtures work and what do not. I have therefore added an appendix, towards the back of this book, that looks at some of the most popular contemporary diets and assesses their compatibility with the principles behind Nic's Keto Diet.

You will find that is perfectly possible to combine Paleo or Atkins with keto, for example, provided you do things properly. But some approaches are much harder to reconcile with my diet. One of them is veganism, which is so important that I am going to say something about it here.

Keto and Veganism

In my experience, combining my (or any other) keto diet with veganism is almost impossible. This is because the sources of protein available to vegans, such as rice and lentils, almost inevitably have high carbohydrate contents.

I tried a no fat, low carb/no sugar diet for a while but to be honest it was hell. You can just about do it if you are a Hindu ascetic eating just one meal a day, but otherwise the combination is likely to be unsustainable for most.

Pescatarianism, on the other hand, is totally compatible with my diet.

Temporary Signs of Ageing

Eventually, you will reach your ideal, 'bottom line' weight. When you get, there, you may notice your face showing signs of ageing. This is only temporary! Drink plenty of water – I get through about four litres/eight pints a day – and eat lots of bone broth. The collagen it contains will help put things right.

Learn to Praise Yourself

Sticking to my diet can be difficult, not because you will feel deprived but because of pressure from outside to join in. One of the best things you can do to combat this is learn to praise yourself. Take pictures of yourself over time and look at them to remind yourself of how far you've come. And treat yourself to some new clothes, which you'll be needing anyway as you lose weight. But keep your old ones for a while before you give them to a charity shop and try them on from time to time. When you feel them sagging, you'll know how well you're doing.

Treats

Many keto diets emphasise the benefits of macadamia nuts. They have a high fat content and are very tasty, but beware: 100g/4oz equates to 700 calories. I would say "it's OK to eat them on a keto diet but don't, because you'll find it very hard to stop at the amount permitted". The same is true of things like honeydew melon and berries. Sure, they're allowed in my diet, but if you eat ten berries, that's your carbohydrate allowance for the day. And are you really capable of stopping at ten?

My philosophy is: don't tease yourself. If you take a tiny lick of a spoon which previously had a sugary desert on it, just to have a taste, you'll simply crave more of it. It isn't worth it. For the same reason, weekly food treats, such as 'keto cakes' (which can certainly be made) are a bad idea. They can easily become an obsession and an expectation.

One treat I do regularly allow myself is 10 to 15g/1/2oz of 99 or 100% cocoa solids chocolate. Once I would have found this too bitter but I love it now. In fact, having retrained my palate, I appreciate all sorts of foods that wouldn't have done anything for me before. Butter, for example, tastes sweet to me now. Nibbling on a pat of it has become a real keto-friendly luxury. I often eat both mine and my wife's when we're given meals on planes.

Cheating

People often ask me if you are allowed the occasional cheat day or cheat meal while you are on my diet. My advice is simple: don't do it. "Once a cheat always a cheat", as they say. Another cliché with a lot of truth in it is "five seconds on your lips, five years on your hips".

I can't deny that I have occasionally cheated while doing my diet, but never for a full day and not at all during the first year. By then I was fat-adapted, which mitigated the damage. I still felt sick though.

Think of it as if you were in a casino and had accumulated a lot of chips. Don't risk losing them just for a transitory moment of pleasure. Life may take away what you have anyway. You may lose that Ferrari you have worked hard for. But leave that to God. Don't throw it away when you have a choice.

What to do When You Plateau

Everyone hits a plateau at some point when dieting. In fact, it is quite likely that this will happen three or four times before you reach your ideal weight.

There are various ways of breaking through a plateau but first you should ask yourself the following questions:

a) Am I keeping my discipline? Am I overeating anything permitted on my diet, e.g. macadamia nuts (100g of which contain about 700 calories)?

b) If I am female, am I having my period or entering the menopause?

c) Am I suffering from an illness?

d) Do I have a mineral deficiency?

e) Have I developed an allergy, for instance to something in my diet?

If the answer to a) is 'yes', it's obvious what to do: restore your discipline and stop eating anything you are indulging in too much! To help you identify where your discipline may be slipping, write down everything you eat and drink for two or three days. And I do mean everything! To keep yourself honest, ask yourself whether you'd be happy to have a camera filming yourself for 24 hours a day to verify what you are eating. Actually, I recommend writing down everything you eat right the way through your diet. It is the best way of spotting when something has gone amiss.

If you suspect the answers to any of b) to e) might be 'yes', consult with your doctor. As I have said before, it is essential to have a good relationship with your GP while you are on this diet.

If you've taken all the above steps and can't find any obvious reason for your weight having plateaued, you have two choices. The first is to be patient and 'sit it out'. Carry on eating what the diet recommends, and your body will eventually comply.

The second option is what I call **Nic's Plateau Buster**. This will break through virtually any weight barrier. Don't do it for more than a week though, or your Omega 3/Omega 6 balance will get out of kilter, causing inflammation problems to set in.

While you are doing the Plateau Buster, you have three meals a day, consisting of the following:

- Three or four eggs (10 total in the day)
- 18g/2/3 oz macadamia nuts OR pine nuts OR sunflower seeds
- 28g/1oz cream cheese

And that is all you eat, for up to a week. You should also take magnesium and vitamin D3 supplements though. After a week, cut out the nuts/seeds and replace with greens.

BMI

Only you can determine the ideal weight for you, but many people use Body Mass Index (BMI) as a guide. This is calculated by dividing your weight in kilograms by the square of your height in metres. A two metre person weighing 100kg would have a BMI of 100 divided by 4, i.e. 25.

The most widely accepted BMI ranges are as follows:

Underweight - less than 18.5

Normal weight – 18.5 to 25

Overweight – 25 to 30

Obese – 30+

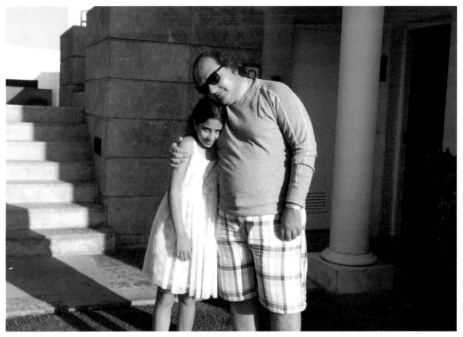

Just started losing weight

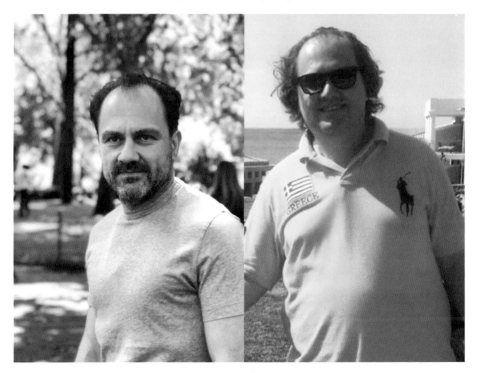

Before and after

4

PART FOUR – THE PROJECT

As I said in Chapter 3, the technical challenge of showing people how to lose weight and live healthier lifestyles through my keto diet is only part of my mission. In a way, this is the easy bit. The greater task is to change the way our societies think about nutrition.

The Study

I am currently doing a PhD entitled 'Evaluation of the effectiveness of "Nic's Keto Diet" vs "Traditional Healthy Diet" in reversing insulin resistance condition in prediabetic and diabetic patients with no other complications.'

While researching various types of diet (high protein, low caloric, different variations of the keto diet), I have established that almost all of them - even the ones that work well in the beginning - have limitations and may cause rebound. This is because they do not treat the main cause of obesity, namely insulin resistance.

On the other hand, I have found that my own keto diet is highly effective when it comes to weight loss, appetite suppression and the enhancement of cognitive and mental functioning.

Our clinical trial aims to prove the effectiveness of Nic's Keto Diet in reversing insulin resistance in pre-diabetic and type 2 diabetes patients, enabling them to lose weight while stopping medication. It also seeks to demonstrate how the diet can improve fatty liver conditions and boost the immune system (specifically, fewer infections and a lowering of the C protein indicators of inflammation).

Another important aspect of the study is an investigation of the effect of my diet on telomeres. These are strands of DNA at the end of our chromosomes that protect them from fraying or sticking to each other. They have often been compared to the plastic tips at the ends of shoelaces. The longer they are, the better. And they can change. This process typically takes four to six months.

One of the most powerful ways of proving the effectiveness of the keto diet would be to show that doing it can increase the length of our telomeres. This would provide objective, incontrovertible evidence.

I wish I'd had my telomeres measured before I started my keto diet. Given my fondness for subjecting myself to medical tests – I may have mentioned that I've done more than 3,000! – this was an unusual omission. But I'm planning to put things right in my PhD. All the participants in the clinical trial will have their telomeres measured both before and after the study.

(Re-) Education and Support

I intend to provide a comprehensive information and support network for people doing my diet.

Mentorship is very helpful for those embarking on my diet, and I am hoping to establish a network of 'keto clinics' to guide them through the process. What I have in mind is somewhat similar to the 'Hope for Health' programme featured in the excellent Netflix film *The Magic Pill*, in which a group of Aboriginal women in Arnhem Land, Northern Australia are reintroduced to their culture's traditional low carb, high protein diet with amazing results.

Social media also has an important role in my plans. As well as spreading the word, it will also help people on the diet to feel part of a community. I want to encourage as many people as possible to test my ideas, in a way reminiscent of crowdfunding, but without the financial commitment. All I will be asking from them is feedback. Whether the diet works for them or not, we need to understand why.

Public Policy

For the keto revolution to make a real difference on a societal level, it is vital to enlist the support of decision makers, opinion-formers, regulatory bodies and so on. That is why I am sending a copy of this book to you!

Change needs to happen at three levels:

The first is political. I believe that politicians already have the correct aim, which is to help people live longer and healthier lives. The problem is that they are working from flawed and outdated data. One of the main purposes of this book is to wake decision makers up to the possibility that the science that has determined dietary policy for the last 50 years or more is wrong. If politicians have the right and duty to prevent us from abusing our bodies with tobacco and drugs, and most of them would claim that they do, I say they have a similar duty to stop us abusing ourselves with sugar.

The second area where change is urgently needed is the field of medical training. As this is my day job, I am in an excellent position to have an influence here.

The final arena where the dominant mentality needs to change is the commercial sector. Businesses are waking up to keto but there is a tendency to try to shortcut the system by promoting what is half-healthy, for example organic foods and nuts, while continuing to add the unnecessary sugar that food producers know make their customers purchase more. I believe that sugar taxes are too little too late, and I would like to see a ban on the funding of medical research by companies with vested interests in the outcome. All too often, for example, the funds for research into diabetes are provided by firms whose business is carbohydrates.

The message I would like to send out to the business community is that I am quite happy to pay more money for less food, as are millions like me.

I understand that politicians are under pressure not to rock the boat by making decisions that threaten vested economic interests. But the fact is that there is no country on Earth that doesn't face problems financing public health. The costs of our excessive consumption of sugars and other carbohydrates are enormous.

In the UK, for example, governments constantly struggle with the issue of how to finance the much-loved but badly overstretched National Health Service. If they put their weight behind the keto diet, the savings would be enormous, because the incidence of 'high carb' diseases would drop dramatically.

To those who claim "we can never overturn the sugar lobby. The businesses involved are simply too powerful", I reply "that's exactly what people said about criticisms of tobacco." I can envisage a future in which governments are sued by their citizens for not warning them about the dangers of high carb diets when they had been scientifically proven.

In the USA, some insurance companies are now paying their customers' subscription costs for an App which guides them through the keto diet, because it saves them so much money through the diseases that are averted.

The American Heart Association putting its sign on products that are low fat and high carb is positively dangerous.

This Book is Only Part One

I want you to think of us as on a journey together. This book is only the start. In due course I will be sending you the results of my PhD study, and more publications are in the pipeline. The keto revolution is gathering momentum and it is going to be exciting discovering what happens next.

A Vision of a Keto Future

I believe that the widespread adoption of a keto-based diet could transform our world. With the incidence of lifestyle diseases falling dramatically, the savings to our beleaguered health systems would be enormous, freeing up funds for other endeavours. Our populations would be healthier, happier, more productive and considerably more mentally alert. There would also be the economic stimulus of a new approach to food production, and many benefits to the environment as the emphasis shifted to organic and grass-fed food.

The day I will know we have succeeded will be when we see a Keto Coke on the shop shelves. This should certainly be possible, with the use of a sweetener such as erythritol or stevia.

I can't wait! (UPDATE – I did actually try one in a small coffee shop a couple of days ago. Now I regret not wishing for something more ambitious!)

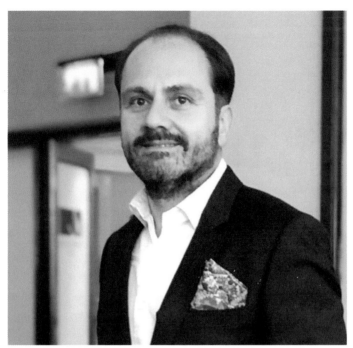

Fat shed like butter in a pan

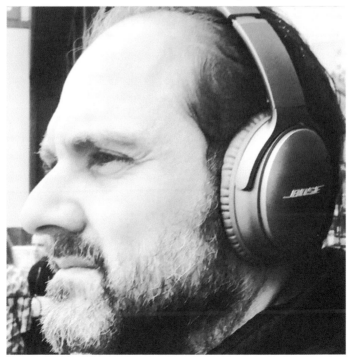

Looking to the bright keto lifestyle

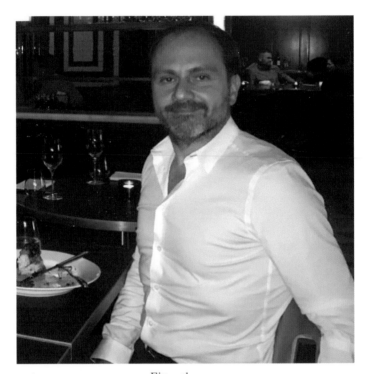

Fitter than ever

CONCLUSION:
THE CHALLENGE

I'm not asking you to take everything I've written at face value. Instead, I'm inviting you to challenge yourself. Ask yourself if what you've been taught about food for all those years really stands up to scrutiny. Consider whether it's possible that our entrenched attitudes to diet have something to do with the epidemics of obesity, diabetes and other modern plagues that are sweeping the planet. And if you feel so moved, why not give my keto diet a try? Then you'll experience the benefits directly, and know what I'm talking about in a way that you never could through words alone.

What have you got to lose?

If I'm wrong, just forget about everything I've said. But if I'm right, and you do nothing about it, you'll be part of the problem. In that case, you will have to bear your share of the responsibility for every life lost due to avoidable insulin resistance.

1

APPENDIX ONE – PEOPLE WHO SHOULD AVOID NIC'S KETO DIET

Below is a fairly comprehensive list of people who should avoid keto.

It is not exhaustive but it's a good starting point. If in any doubt, please consult your doctor. Anyone planning to embark on my diet is advised to do this first.

People suffering from any of the following conditions should not go on my diet:

- Type 1 diabetes
- Symptoms of addiction to alcohol, food and drugs
- Previously diagnosed cancers, or polyps of the intestines and colon
- Previous or current pathology of the pancreas
- Carnitine deficiency (primary)
- Carnitine palmitoyltransferase (CPT) I or II deficiency
- Carnitine translocase deficiency
- Beta-oxidation defects

- Mitochondrial 3-hydroxy-3-methylglutaryl-CoA synthase (mHMGS) deficiency
- Medium-chain acyl dehydrogenase deficiency (MCAD)
- Long-chain acyl dehydrogenase deficiency (LCAD)
- Short-chain acyl dehydrogenase deficiency (SCAD)
- Long-chain 3-hydroxyacyl-CoA deficiency
- Medium-chain 3-hydroxyacyl-CoA deficiency
- Pyruvate carboxylase deficiency
- Porphyria

2

APPENDIX TWO – SOURCES OF FURTHER INFORMATION

The keto community of scientists, dieticians and trainers is constantly growing, but there are a few people who have been a special inspiration to me. I strongly recommend that you look at some of their work.

Dr Jason Fung:

Dr Fung is a Canadian nephrologist, who lives and works in Toronto. He's a world-leading expert on intermittent fasting and low carb dieting, especially for treating people with type 2 diabetes. He has written three best-selling health books and is a co-founder of the Intensive Dietary Management program.

Website and Blog: idm.program.com

Dr Eric Westman:

Dr Westman MD, MHS, Chief Medical Officer, is Associate Professor of Medicine at Duke University. He is Chairman of the Board of the Obesity Medicine Association, a Fellow of the Obesity Society and a co-editor of a medical textbook on obesity.

He is the author of the New York Times bestseller The New Atkins for a New You.

Dr Eric Berg:

A health educator specialising in weight loss through natural, nutritional methods, Dr Berg is one of the world's top keto diet experts. His clients include senior U.S. Government officials, ambassadors, doctors, high-level executives of prominent corporations, scientists, professors, and others from all walks of life.

His website, www.drberg.com, is an excellent keto resource.

Thomas Delauer:

An American celebrity trainer, entrepreneur and author, Delauer is well known for his writings on inflammation in the human body. He was a passionate exerciser in his youth, but lost his muscular physique when he took time away from the gym to concentrate on business. Then he got it back again, and now helps others to do the same.

See www.greatestphysiques.com/thomas-delauer/

Professor Tim Noakes:

Tim Noakes is Emeritus Professor in the Division of Exercise Science and Sports Medicine at the University of Cape Town . He is a champion of a low-carb, high fat diet, and has successfully defended it in the courts in the face of attacks from the South African medical establishment.

He is a real hero of mine and my prayers are with him. His books include *The Real Meal Revolution* and *Lore of Nutrition: Challenging Conventional Dietary Beliefs.*

The Magic Pill *(Netflix):*

Mainstream TV has largely ignored the keto movement but this excellent and fascinating documentary is an exception.

3

APPENDIX THREE – MEASURING YOUR KETONE LEVELS

To do my diet effectively, or any keto diet for that matter, you absolutely have to know whether you are in a state of ketosis or not. If you are not, you will need to adjust your food consumption until you are.

It is also extremely interesting to see exactly how what you eat, how long you leave between meals and what exercise you do affects the ketone levels in your bloodstream. This information will put you in control of what is happening in your body, which is exactly the point of my diet.

There are three main ways of measuring your ketone levels. None of them is free but what price can you put on your health?

Blood Testing for BHB (beta-Hydroxybutyric acid)

This method involves pricking your finger to obtain a small drop of blood, which you place on a test strip. This is then analysed by a hand-held machine, which measures the level of

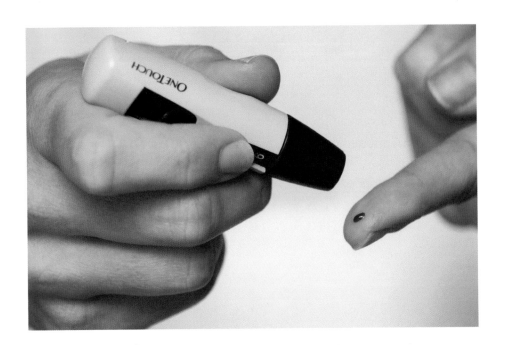

BHB in your blood. This is the predominant ketone in your body.

The procedure is very like that carried out by diabetics several times per day. In fact, identical monitoring machines can be used - many of them can be set to measure either BHB or blood glucose levels, depending on the kind of test strips employed.

Equipment needed:
- Hand-held measuring device (e.g. Precision Xtra or Keto Mojo)
- Ketone test strips
- Lancets
- Alcohol (for swabbing your finger before and after testing)

Pros:

- Gives the most accurate results of the three methods mentioned here
- Tests for BHB, which is far more prevalent in the blood than the other main ketone bodies acetoacetate or acetone

Cons:

- Some people find obtaining blood samples by pricking their fingers unpleasant until they get used to it
- Relatively expensive. A complete kit, consisting of monitor, lancets, test strips etc. will set you back around £45/$60. Replacement test strips are around 80p/$1 each

Urine Tests

This is a cheaper and less invasive way of testing your ketone levels. The downside is that it measures acetoacetate, which gives a less reliable reading than BHB testing.

Pros:

- Cheap
- Easy and non-invasive
- Strips readily available from pharmacies

Cons:

• Measures acetoacetates rather than BHBs

• Indicates what your body is excreting, not what is in your bloodstream. As you become keto-adapted, you will expel fewer ketone bodies in your urine as your system becomes better at using them as fuel. At this point, the test may suggest your ketone levels are dropping when this isn't the case at all

• This method can give very different results depending on your hydration levels. This can be misleading

Breath acetone meter

One way you can tell if you are in ketosis is if your breath smells of acetone – the substance that gives nail varnish its distinctive smell. This method makes use of the fact that ketosis leaves an imprint on your breath.

Pros:

• Easiest, most convenient method

• One-off cost. Once you have bought a monitoring device (typically for around £175/$250), this method is essentially free

• Although acetone is not the most prevalent ketone in the body, research indicates that the readings obtained through this method relate well to actual levels of ketone bodies in the blood, at least at low concentrations

Cons:

- Initial outlay is high
- Not as accurate as blood tests

4

APPENDIX FOUR – COMPARISON OF NIC'S KETO DIET WITH OTHER POPULAR CONTEMPORARY DIETS

I am not so biased as to assume that keto is the only important diet out there, or the only one that works. I am also well aware, as I mentioned on page 98, that people often get the best results by combining elements from different diets. This section, therefore, looks at the pros and cons of several popular contemporary diets, and considers whether they are keto-compatible.

Atkins

Overview:
Developed by Dr Robert Atkins during the 1960s, this is arguably the most famous low carbohydrate diet in the world. Like the Keto diet, it is based on the principle that if you heavily restrict carbohydrate intake, your body will start burning fat.

The Atkins diet has four 'phases'. During the first, you may not consume more than 20g of net carbs per day. Pasta, grains, bread and potatoes are banned, as are nuts, seeds, legumes, pulses, caffeine and alcohol. In the second 'balancing' phase, net carb intake is increased by 5g per day until it reaches 50g. Low carb fruit, grains and vegetables and alcoholic drinks are gradually reintroduced. More carbohydrates are slowly introduced slowly during phases three and four, until you reach the 'maintenance' level of 100g per day, at which your weight is supposed to stabilise.

In its original form, the Atkins diet did not distinguish sufficiently between 'good' and 'bad' kinds of fat and protein but this was subsequently put right.

Pros:

It is possible to lose weight very quickly, particularly during phase one.

The basic concept is simple and clear.

Cons:

Many people experience side effects during the early phases, including bad breath, tiredness and constipation, the latter caused by a sudden reduction in fibre intake.

As mentioned on page 47, Doctor Atkins did not fully appreciate the potential for excess protein to be converted into body fat.

Foods You Can Eat:

Meat, seafood, eggs, dairy products, nuts, fats, oils

Foods to Avoid:

Fruits and vegetables (in early phases), grains, legumes, sugar, honey

Compatibility with NKD:

High, provided a lid is kept on the quantity of protein consumed. The addition of the cruciferous vegetables and MCT oil in Nic's Keto Diet will help tackle the side effects.

South Beach

Overview:

Originally developed for heart patients in the USA by the cardiologist Dr Arthur Agatston and the dietician Marie Almon, the South Beach diet is a lower-fat alternative to the Atkins diet.

There is no calorie counting and no limit on portion size. You eat three meals and two snacks a day, and are encouraged to follow an exercise plan.

The diet has three phases. During the first, which lasts for two weeks, you eat lean meat, vegetables with a low glycemic index (i.e. ones which do not raise blood sugar levels dramatically) and unsaturated fats. Weight loss is expected to be rapid – up to 6kg/13.2lbs. In the second phase, carbs with a low glycemic index are gradually reintroduced. Phase three is all about maintenance.

Pros:

The absence of calorie counting or limits on portion size will appeal to many.

Rapid weight loss during phase 1.

After phase 1, all the major food groups are included in the diet, which will keep your doctor happy.

Cons:

You can expect to experience similar side effects to people on the Atkins diet, particularly in phase 1.

Foods You Can Eat:

Meat, seafood, dairy products, eggs, nuts, fats, ols, non-starchy vegetables, legumes

Foods to Avoid:

Fruit, grains, legumes, sugar, honey

Compatibility with NKD:

High, with similar caveats to those that apply to the Atkins diet

Paleo

Overview:

Also known as the caveman diet, Paleo is based on the presumed eating habits of our ancestors before the dawn of agriculture around 10,000 years ago. It is based around foods that can be hunted, fished and gathered. Cereal grains, dairy products, potatoes, refined sugar and all processed foods are excluded.

There is no official Paleo diet but all versions are low carb and high protein. More research is needed to assess its weight loss potential, which is obviously going to depend on the quantities of food consumed.

Pros:

The ban on processed foods automatically removes many unhealthy substances from the diet.

Intuitively makes sense – many of humanity's health and other problems began with the development of agriculture.

Likely to appeal to people with conditions like gluten-intolerance.

Cons:

We don't actually know what our distant ancestors ate, nor how healthy they typically were.

Omission of certain food groups can lead to vitamin deficiencies.

Foods You Can Eat:
Meat, seafood, eggs, nuts, oils, non-starchy vegetables and fruit.

Foods to Avoid:
Anything processed, dairy products, grains, beans and sugar.

Compatibility with NKD:
High, given careful portion control and limits on protein intake.

Mediterranean

Overview:
The Mediterranean diet focuses on the traditional eating habits of Southern Europeans, particularly in Crete, other parts of Greece, and southern Italy. It is the most extensively studied diet of all and has been shown to lower the risk of numerous diseases, including cardiovascular ones.

The diet emphasises simple, unprocessed foods, with abundant vegetables and fruits, and plenty of cheese and yoghurt. Olive oil is the main source of dietary fat. Cheese and yogurts are the most important dairy foods, and fish and poultry may be consumed in moderation, along with a small amount of red meat. Up to a third of the Mediterranean diet consists of fat, most of it unsaturated.

Pros:

This is a healthy and balanced diet, and people in the relevant parts of the Mediterranean can live for a very long time.

Studies have shown that the Mediterranean diet can significantly the risk of developing cardiovascular disease and type 2 diabetes.

Cons:

This isn't a particularly good diet for those seeking rapid weight loss.

Foods You Can Eat:

Meat, seafood (particularly fatty and oily fish), nuts, fats, oils (particularly extra virgin olive oil), non-starchy greens, low card fruits and wine! (In moderation).

Foods to Avoid:

Processed foods, starchy vegetables, rice, sugar and high carb fruits.

Compatibility with NKD:

Medium to High, if the beans and grains are cut out and care is taken to align the diet with your macros (see page 70).

Zone

Overview:

The Zone diet was developed by Dr Barry Sears to minimise his patients' risk of inflammation. He believes that excessive blood sugar is a major cause of this problem. The 'Zone' referred to in the name is the steady blood sugar level that the diet seeks to achieve.

People on the Zone diet eat five times a day – three main meals and two snacks – and the food they consume is 30% protein, 40% carbohydrate and 30% 'good' fat.

Pros:

The Zone diet is extremely precise, which will appeal to some people.

Provided you stick to the prescribed ratios, you have great flexibility about what you eat.

The emphasis on reducing inflammation is healthy and in tune with my own approach.

Cons:

The need to stick to the 30/40/30 ratio can make dining out tricky.

More research is needed on the effectiveness of the diet.

Foods You Can Eat:
Anything, in moderate quantities.

Foods to Avoid:
None.

Compatibility with NKD:
Low, largely because the prescribed protein/carbohydrate/ fat ratios and the 'anything goes' approach are very different.

Vegan

Overview
Veganism is arguably more of a philosophy that a diet. It is based on the avoidance of all animal-based products, including dairy products, eggs and honey.

Pros:
Environmental friendliness and compassion for animals.

Avoidance of growth hormones and other unpleasant additives frequently used in meat production.

Cons:
Care must be taken to avoid nutritional deficiencies.

Foods You Can Eat:
Anything not animal-based.

Foods to Avoid:

All animal-based products.

Compatibility with NKD:

Low. It is extremely difficult to achieve ketosis while eating a vegan diet, as the available sources of protein such as pulses and rice are invariably high in sugar (see page 99).

Weight Watchers

Overview:

The Weight Watchers programme is all about controlling calorie intake. It is based on a points system, which gives foods and drinks values according to their carbohydrate, protein, fat and fibre contents. Each participant has a daily points allowance. How they use it is up to them.

Some foods, like fruits and most vegetables, are rated zero, which means you can eat as much of them as you wish.

The goal is steady weight loss, at a rate of around 1kg/2lbs per week.

Pros:

Weekly meetings and confidential weigh-ins provide vital emotional support.

The points system educates you about calorie values.

Encourages a measured and steady approach to weight loss.

Cons:

The freedom to eat anything you want makes you very vulnerable to temptation and bad habits. It also means that you are likely to consume things that spike your blood sugar.

The point system can be difficult and time-consuming, particularly for newcomers.

Weight loss is relatively slow.

Foods You Can Eat:

Any, provided you remain within your points allowance.

Foods to Avoid:

None, provided you remain within your points allowance.

Compatibility with NKD:

Very low. While I know it has worked for some, I would advise against this kind of diet.

5:2 Intermittent Fasting

Overview

There are many forms of intermittent fasting. One of the most popular is the 5:2 diet, in which you eat normally for five days of the week and fast on the other two. The definition of 'fasting' is rather loose though – women are allowed to consume 500 calories and men 600.

Pros:

The 'fasting' days provide many of the benefits associated with genuine fasting (see page 65).

The rules of the 5:2 diet are extremely simple.

Many people find restricting food intake for just two days a week much easier than doing it for seven.

The rules are simple to follow.

Cons:

May tempt you to over-eat on non-fasting days.

Not suitable for pregnant women, diabetics and people with eating disorders.

Foods You Can Eat:

Any, provided you 'fast' for two days a week.

Foods to Avoid:

None, provided you fast for two days a week.

Compatibility with NKD:

Mixed. Low in the sense that you can eat all sorts of things that are not permitted on my diet. High in the emphasis on the benefits of intermittent fasting.

Raw Food

Overview:

As the name implies, the raw food diet is based on the consumption of uncooked food. Adherents believe that at least 75% of a person's food intake should not have been cooked. Raw food can be defined as that has not been refined, chemically processed or canned, and has not been heated above 48C. The significance of this figure is that at higher temperatures, many of the natural enzymes present in food are destroyed.

Raw foodists can be vegetarian, vegan or carnivorous. There are even fruitarians, who only eat fruit, with the addition of nuts and/or seeds for the less strict.

Pros:

Versatility, provided the 'raw' clause is obeyed.

Avoids many harmful chemicals used in or created by food processing.

Raw food is typically higher in vitamins and other nutrients than the cooked equivalent.

Cons:

Bloating and gas can be problematic side effects.

Rules out a lot of meat and fish dishes.

Foods You Can Eat:

Virtually anything, provided it is raw.

Foods to Avoid:

Anything that has been refined, chemically processed, canned or heated above 48C.

Compatibility with NKD:

Medium. It is certainly possible to combine a raw food diet with my approach, provided care is taken to consume enough protein and fat. Sashimi can be very helpful here.

Low Fat

Overview

Low fat diets used to be the default approach to losing weight, partly due to the efforts of people like Ancel Keys (see page 43). But as I have emphasised in this book, the demonisation of fat has caused all kinds of problems.

There can be no more persuasive argument for avoiding this kind of diet than the dramatic decline in health of the general population while it was the dominant approach. I STRONGLY ADVISE AGAINST LOW FAT DIETS.

Pros:

Fats contain more calories (nine per gram) than carbohydrates (four per gram). Other things being equal, therefore, reducing fat intake is a more effective way of losing weight than eating fewer carbs. But other things are not equal. To repeat what I said at the beginning of this book, biology is not simple mathematics. Our bodies break down what we eat and turn it into other things, including energy. AVOIDING FAT DOESN'T AUTOMATICALLY LEAD TO WEIGHT LOSS, NOR CONSUMING IT TO WEIGHT GAIN.

Cons:

Low fat diets are terrible at making you feel full. They can also lack flavour. As a consequence, you will almost inevitably eat more carbohydrates than you should to compensate. This will cause all sorts of problems highlighted elsewhere in this book, like insulin resistance.

A diet that is too low in fat can prevent you absorbing fat-soluble vitamins properly (A, D, E and K). It can also be harmful to brain functioning, which absolutely relies on fats.

Foods You Can Eat:

Ones with low fat content.

Foods to Avoid:

High fat foods.

Compatibility with NKD:

Extremely poor. AVOID.

5

APPENDIX FIVE – ESSENTIALS OF MY DIET

Coffee

To be honest, even I would find it difficult to do my diet without coffee. It makes you feel full and wards off hunger pangs. It also keeps you energised to spend more of your reserve calories.

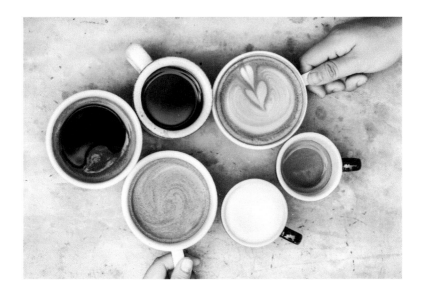

There are only two potential downsides. First, it isn't a good idea to consume too much caffeine, so when you've had enough, just drunk your coffee decaf. Secondly, caffeine does induce some insulin reaction. The solution to this is Keto Coffee – the regular drink with MCT oil added. I can't recommend this highly enough.

Matcha Tea

An even better thing to drink while on my diet is matcha – the powdered green tea from Japan used in the famous tea ceremony. High in vitamins, it is also rich in antioxidants. One of them, a catechin called EGCg, is widely recognised for its cancer fighting properties and has even been found to help people lose weight.

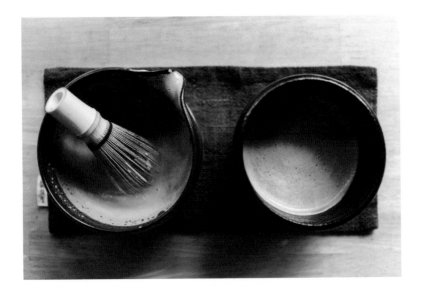

Eggs

Nothing can beat eggs on Nic's Keto Diet. They keep you full and balanced, and can rightly be described as a 'super food'.

When you consider the function of an egg, and the yolk in particular, this isn't surprising. It has to provide everything a baby bird needs to grow from a single cell organism into a creature ready for the outside world.

Egg yolk contains thirteen essential vitamins and minerals, plus the eye-protecting antioxidants lutein and zeaxanthin. It is also one of the best sources of choline, an essential vitamin-like nutrient that is involved in many vital physiological processes.

Although egg yolks are high in cholesterol, eating them doesn't raise blood cholesterol levels in most people. Indeed, they have been been shown to modify Low Density Lipoproteins (LDLs) in a way that reduces the risk of heart disease.

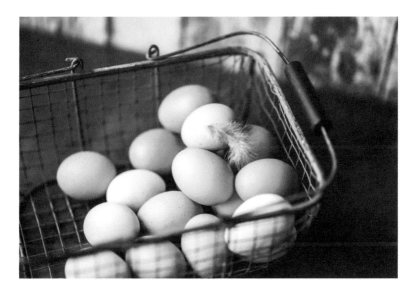

The consumption of eggs has been demonstrated to enhance feelings of fullness and to keep blood sugar levels stable. This helps you to eat fewer calories. And one large egg contains fewer than 6g of protein and less than 1 gram of carbohydrate. It is the perfect keto-friendly food.

Avocados

Oily, rich and delicious, avocados are an essential part of the keto diet. They are especially useful in the early stages, because of their high vitamin and mineral content. The potassium in them helps prevent the symptoms of keto flu and they are a much better option for this than the high-carb banana.

In the long term, avocados have beneficial effects on cholesterol and triglyceride levels. One study found that an increased consumption of avocados led to a 22% decrease in

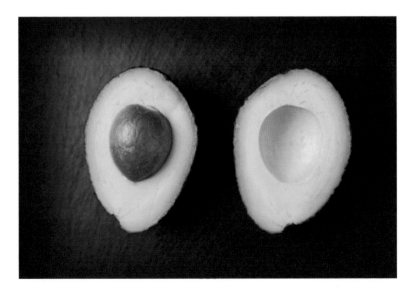

'bad' LDL cholesterol and an 11% increase in 'good' HDL cholesterol.

A medium-sized avocado contains about 18g of carbohydrates, but 14 of these are made up of fibre. About two thirds of this is insoluble, meaning that it passes out of your system undigested.

Apple Cider Vinegar

All sorts of extravagant claims are made for the benefits of apple cider vinegar. What is undoubtedly true is that it makes an extremely valuable contribution to my keto diet.

Among its most beneficial effects, apple cider vinegar can lower blood sugar levels and combat diabetes. Studies have shown it to improve insulin sensitivity during a high-carb meal by 19–34%, and to reduce blood sugar by 34% after the

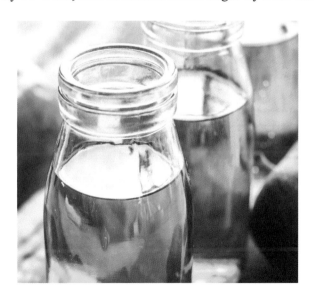

consumption of 50g/2oz of white bread.

Amazingly, apple cider can also help you to lose weight, particularly belly fat. One three-month study of 175 obese subjects found that those who ate a tablespoonful per day lost an average of 1.2kg/2.6kg, while those who took 2 tbs per day lost 1.7kg/3.7lbs.

I wouldn't advise people to consume much more than 2tbs per day, but even at that level it can have remarkable effects. You can either use it in salad dressings, homemade mayonnaise etc, or drink it diluted with water.

Cruciferous Vegetables

Also known as brassicas, these dark, leafy vegetables are the main addition of my diet to 'standard keto'. Only avocados and spinach beat them in importance.

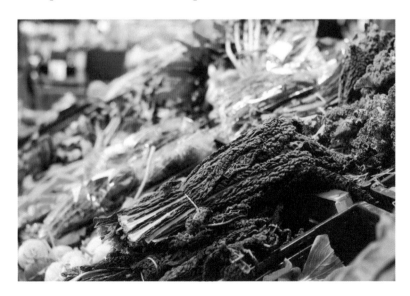

They include broccoli, cabbage, bok choy, collard greens, brussels sprouts and kale. Cabbage is best eaten in its fermented form as sauerkraut and kale should be eaten in moderation as it has a high sugar content.

One of the most valuable contributions of cruciferous vegetables to my diet is that they help maintain the potassium balance in your body. Without this essential mineral, you will find it very difficult to lose weight.

Sleep

Getting enough sleep is extremely important when doing my diet. I would describe eight hours as mandatory.

Of course, sleep is vital to good health anyway. It reboots your metabolism and plays a vital role in helping your body to fight off disease. Meta-analysis of 16 separate studies covering more than 1.3 million people over a period of 25 years found that subjects who generally slept for less than six hours a night were 12% more likely to die prematurely. Meanwhile, reducing sleep time from seven hours to five or less has been shown to increase the chances of dying from any cause by 70 % in the long term.

These are excellent reasons to make sure you get enough sleep but it becomes particularly important when you are dieting.

One reason for this is that too little sleep causes stress, which raises your levels of cortisol. As I mentioned on page

91, this makes it very difficult to lose weight, as the hormone is essentially an instruction to your body to hold on to its energy reserves.

Another factor is that sleep helps you manage your appetite. It shortens the waking period without food, and obviously you won't be eating when you're asleep, unless you're an expert somnambulist! Poor sleeping habits increase the body's energy needs, and when you are sleep-deprived, your brain will release chemicals to signal hunger. This is likely to cause you to eat more, and thus to gain weight.

Researchers conducting a study of almost 5,000 Japanese adults with type 2 diabetes found that those who slept fewer than 4.5 hours or more than 8.5 (excessive sleep isn't good either) hours had higher BMIs and blood sugar levels.

There are lots of books and plenty of information online about how to improve your sleeping habits. What I will say here is that you should avoid the blue light emitted by computer screens and television for a couple of hours before you go to bed. And if you find it difficult to get enough good quality sleep, magnesium supplements can be helpful.

6

APPENDIX SIX – FASTING IN DIFFERENT RELIGIOUS AND CULTURAL TRADITIONS

Intermittent fasting is an important aspect of Nic's Keto Diet. It isn't compulsory – you can obtain many of the benefits of my diet without doing it - but it will make a huge difference to your physical and spiritual well-being.

The purpose of this section is to show just how prevalent the practice of fasting has been in history, and how deeply embedded it is in many of our cultures.

Christianity

The most demanding form of fasting in the Christian tradition is the so-called Black Fast. It was strictly adhered to by all denominations up until the late Middle Ages, particularly during Lent. Nowadays, only certain religious groups practice it.

The Black Fast had the following rules:
- Only one meal per day allowed
- It had to be eaten after sunset
- The consumption of meat, eggs, dairy products and alcohol were forbidden
- During Holy Week, the only things you could eat were bread, herbs, salt and water

Eastern Orthodoxy

In the tradition in which I grew up, the Black Fast is still observed during Lent. Similar fasts are also practiced during Advent, the two weeks prior to the Dormition of Mary on August 15th, and for between 8 and 42 days prior to the Feast of Saints Peter and Paul on 29th June.

Roman Catholicism

The Black Fast used to be strictly observed during Lent, and by trainee priests in the run-up to their ordination.

Today, Roman Catholics who are fasting are permitted to eat two small 'collations' in addition to the main meal of the day, provided that the combined quantity of food eaten in both is less than they consume during the latter.

Catholics are also required to refrain from eating for at least an hour before taking Holy Communion.

The Eastern Catholics, who are in full communion with

the Pope but do not use the Latin rite, are stricter about fasting, eating only one meal during the day and avoiding animal products.

Anglicanism

During the 19th Century, the Black Fast was widely practiced on Ash Wednesday and Good Friday.

Pentecostalism

There are no set days for fasting within the Classical Pentecostalist calendar, but members of the congregation are positively expected to receive guidance from the Holy Spirt to fast from time to time.

In Pentecostalist circles, a Black Fast is complete abstinence from food or water, although the church authorities teach that such fasts should be undertaken for more than three successive days because of health risks.

In practice, Pentecostalists usually observe what they call 'Normal Fasts', in which only pure water may be consumed.

Mormonism

Mormons traditionally abstain from two meals on the first Sunday of every month. During their fast, they share personal testimonies with other members of the community.

Islamism

Fasting, or Sawm, is one of the Five Pillars of Islam, along with charity, Shahada (the declaration of faith), prayer five times daily, and the Hajj pilgrimage to Mecca.

The most important ritual fasting takes place during the month of Ramadan. Food and drink may not be consumed during daylight hours, and sexual relations are forbidden.

The idea is to abstain from all bodily pleasures to develop self-control, better understanding of the gifts of Allah (God) and more compassion for the deprived.

Various groups are exempted from the fast, including pre-pubescent children, the sick, women who are pregnant, breastfeeding or menstruating, and people who are travelling.

Judaism

Fasting for observant Jews means completely abstaining from food and drink, water included.

There are six fasting days in the traditional Jewish calendar. On two of them, Yom Kippur and Tisha B'Av, washing the body, wearing leather, using perfume and having sex are also forbidden. Fasting is forbidden, however, on Shabbat (the Sabbath), as the biblical commandment to observe it is held to override other considerations.

Some Jewish fasts run from sunset to sunset, others from dawn until the appearance of stars in the evening.

Buddhism

The primary purpose of fasting in Buddhism is the development of self-control. Prior to attaining enlightenment, Siddhartha Gutama, the founder of Buddhism, practiced extreme asceticism for a period, eating very little food, but he did not advocate this for his followers. Instead, he recommended the 'Middle Path' of moderation. He did, however, advise monks and nuns not to eat after their midday meal, which is effectively a form of intermittent fasting.

Lay Buddhists are encouraged to follow the same practice on Uposatha ('observance') days, which occur about once a week in parts of the world where Theravada Buddhism is practiced, and more frequently in Mahayana countries.

Hinduism

Fasting is an extremely important aspect of traditional Hindu religious observance, though the ways in which it is practiced vary a great deal according to geographical location and between individuals.

The fundamental purpose of fasting for Hindus is to deny the physical desires of the body, thus focusing the mind on what really matters – the spiritual dimension. A strict fast entails consuming no food or water from sunset of day one until precisely 48 minutes after sunrise on day three, approximately 36 hours later.

Common rituals include strict fasting or avoiding certain foods like fish or meat on certain days every month, during festivals or on the day of the week associated with the deity to which the individual is specially devoted. Devotees of Shiva tend to fast on Mondays, for example, and followers of Vishnu on Thursdays.

THANKS AND ACKNOWLEDGEMENTS

This journey would not have been possible without the unlimited support of my precious wife Natalia. She has shared my ups and downs, my lean, fat and very fat days. She was the one light that blinked hope when fatty depression struck, and made the cravings, doubts and external criticism just seem like passages to her warm, welcoming arms. This amazing, loving creature knows how to balance her worries - that my diet goes against the usual crazy low-fat theories diet she was taught – with her constant support for my journey on keto. If the ideal of my diet is a healthier, longer life, the prize is her wonderful smile when she sees that I'm making it happen. Thank you for everything Natasha.

Special thanks go to my sisters Dr Mary (MD) and Zalfa (psychologist), my brother Marwan, and their husbands and spouses (Dr Tony, Dr Ara, Corine), and to my dearest nieces and nephew: Christina, Perla, Christa-Maria, Julia, Christy

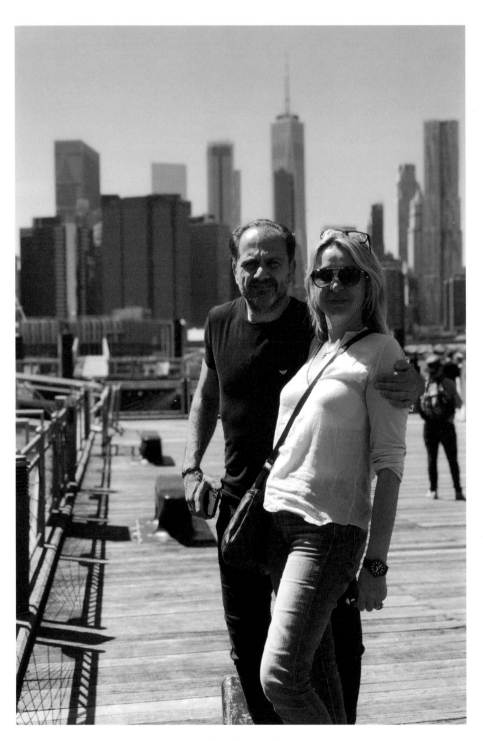

Me and my wife

and Marco, my supportive egg-eater and vacation and gym companion. Their pride in their fit uncle means the world to me. They have always done everything to make me feel comfortable, even when they have worried about the possible excesses of my diet. Now I need their support to help change the world.

Thank you dad (Elie), for always supporting my dreams, even when you did not believe in them. You taught me the value of doubt, and scientific doubt is what makes new discoveries possible.

My prayers are for my mum Alice. Her angel did not leave me alone on my journey to be better, and her prayers safeguard me from wrong doing and wrong thought. Her love still fuels my passion to go further whenever the road is hard. Mum, I made it! I am fit and slim but not skinny. Your wish became true.

GOD Bless the soul of my uncle Elias, the man who sponsored my early education and inspired me to believe that success is the certain result of hard work and honesty. You were always there when needed and you knew how to shield your family from life's hard times, as well as how to enjoy the good ones.

Thank you to my Uncles , Aunts, to my cousins, wider family, friends and every person who encouraged me with full love and hope.

Huge thanks to my NKD Team, especially but not limited

to Dr Ghassan, the support stone who can hold any project together through his devotion and hard work.

A special 'thank you' to Sergey, our nephew and future project developer, whose talk about macros was the inspiration for the start of the journey, and our new partners, who have hopped onto the bus but are really ready for the driver's seat. Dear NKD Team, your help and support remain essential to make this the world's way of dieting and living a healthier life.

Thank you to my brothers in spirit, Dr Chahine (MD). Dr Chahine Mohammad, your support is invaluable you are always there at all times and circumstances when your support is essential to make it happen.

Thank you to Kursk State Medical University, to the visionary rector, professors, teachers and staff who have made my life worth living. The thousands of doctors we have trained are making the world a healthier place to live in. With your help, maybe one day keto will be part of mainstream medicine.

See you all soon with the results of our trials and more keto success stories!

Nicolas@trccolleges.com
www.ketoandorganic.com

31605493R00095

Printed in Poland
by Amazon Fulfillment
Poland Sp. z o.o., Wrocław